About

Dr James Fleming is an Accident and
Emergency doctor at Preston Royal Infirmary.
He studied at Manchester University and has
worked in obstetrics, gynaecology and
general medicine, and in ophthalmology in
Adelaide, Australia. He writes a weekly
column on medical issues for the *Craven
Herald and Pioneer* and *Beat Cellulite Forever* is
his first book. He lives in Chorley.

Beat
CELLULITE
forever

Beat
CELLULITE
forever

What works
What doesn't

DR JAMES FLEMING

PIATKUS

Visit the Piatkus website!

Piatkus publishes a wide range of best-selling fiction and non-fiction, including books on health, mind, body & spirit, sex, self-help, cookery, biography and the paranormal.

If you want to:
- read descriptions of our popular titles
- buy our books over the internet
- take advantage of our special offers
- enter our monthly competition
- learn more about your favourite Piatkus authors

VISIT OUR WEBSITE AT: www.piatkus.co.uk

Copyright © 2002 by James Fleming

First published in 2002 by
Judy Piatkus (Publishers) Limited
5 Windmill Street
London W1T 2JA
e-mail: info@piatkus.co.uk

Reprinted 2002

The moral right of the author has been asserted

A catalogue record for this book is available from the British Library

ISBN 0–7499–2281-8

This book has been printed on paper manufactured with respect for the environment using wood from managed sustainable resources

Text design by Paul Saunders

Typeset by Phoenix Photosetting, Chatham, Kent
Printed and bound in Great Britain by
Mackays Ltd, Chatham, Kent

Note for Readers

The information presented in this book has been accumulated from medical journals, training, patients, beauty salons and personal experience. It is important that the reader understands that these guidelines are not intended to be prescriptive, nor are they an attempt to diagnose any specific condition.

Recommendations contained within the text are based on the author's research and experience. His views are completely independent. He is not employed by any pharmaceutical company, medical journal, food supplement supplier or food company.

It is recommended that you tell your medical adviser of any dietary changes, exercise regimes or food supplement programmes you intend to follow. Obtain as much information as possible about any of the treatments in this book before following them. The list of side-effects may not be comprehensive in this book. Some of the treatments may interfere with a treatment from your doctor that you are already taking.

Note also that medical science is changing so fast that a treatment may have changed by the time this book is published.

Disclaimer

Contents

Introduction

THE RESEARCH FOR THIS book has been a long, but enjoyable journey. There seemed to be a never-ending supply of information about cellulite from countless different sources. What started as a simple compendium of the information about cellulite became a huge undertaking.

I have been asked many times by patients, friends and family if I know of a cure for cellulite. My answer was always vague because I did *not* know. After reading about the subject on the internet I realised that all the information I was finding contained no proof. The statements about the causes of cellulite and the treatment of cellulite were not backed up by any evidence. This was when I decided to write a book on the subject.

Everything I do in clinical practice is under the closest scrutiny. All the drugs and treatments that I prescribe have been regulated by the country's drug authorities. When people are treated by me they know that I am accountable for my actions and they know that anything I prescribe, should it cause them adverse side-effects, is covered under the umbrella of litigation should they wish to pursue that. This is because our social system provides the public with protection from adverse reactions to treatment by the NHS.

The same is not true for the treatment of cellulite. This is not recognised by the medical profession in that there is no established set of treatment options for it. Cellulite is the *appearance* of fat and is used as a colloquial term to describe this. There are ways of describing it medically that I explain later in the book. It is not seen as a disease, so the treatments available are usually ones that have to be paid for. In order to have cosmetic treatment on the NHS you have to demonstrate that the condition in question, say small breasts, is making you depressed to the point where it needs changing to save your sanity. That is very hard to do.

As the treatments for cellulite have to be paid for, the door is open for anyone to start selling things that are claimed to treat cellulite. These treatments do not have to be regulated if they are sold directly to the customer and if the vendor works for no professional body.

There is also no need to list the ingredients of a treatment on the side of the box, nor its possible side-effects, so a lot of the time you do not know what you are buying or what the side-effects may be. Even in a beauty salon it is only necessary to claim that a treatment for cellulite works for it to be sold as such.

After collating the information on all the types of cellulite treatments available I had to find out whether they worked or not. There is some direct evidence to say that some of these treatments do work, based on the results of lengthy clinical trials that took place in hospitals. Some of the treatments have not been studied formally but working around the information that is available it was possible to say whether they might work based on logic and physiology. There are some treatments that, however I look at them, I cannot see how they can work for the treatment of cellulite.

The media today bombards us with photographs of perfect people that make all of us feel physically inadequate at some time in our lives. Women see 15-year old, 6 foot models on the pages of magazines and believe that to be the norm. This is one of the main reasons behind our current obsession with cellulite and why so many people are spending large sums of money on treatments. They may think that they have been having treatment for cellulite for many years so they should see some benefit. That is not necessarily the case. If the treatment does not work, then it has been wasted money. If it does work yet it has not been proven to, then fine. If you are planning to try a new treatment, or there seems to be no results from a current treatment, then this book is for you. This will allow you to see the basis for its use as a cellulite treatment and you can make up your own mind about whether to carry on the treatment or not.

We are troubled by many diseases these days largely because we are tending to live longer. We suffer from headaches, sleep problems, stress, stomach cramps, obesity. We work too hard, try to fit too much into one lifetime, eat badly, take little exercise and drink too much. The short answer for many people is to start looking for pills to take, for instance, food supplements or fast cures for cellulite in the form of a potion. I would like people to know what they are buying in the field of cellulite treatments, particularly with this being my chosen specialist subject. We have enough to cope with without the threat of taking a pill that might cause us to be ill.

Beat Cellulite Forever is a brand new, comprehensive approach that includes all the latest treatments for cellulite, together with plenty of useful tips for a healthier lifestyle.

There are no hard regimes in this book. It is especially easy to follow, needs no specialist knowledge and will allow women to make an informed choice about one aspect of their bodies.

Why write another cellulite book?

There are many books out there on dieting, exercise, detoxification and cellulite. It has been my intention to use the knowledge that I have gained from being a doctor to contribute to this field. As a doctor I have been taught that a patient has to make an informed choice about his or her treatment. Over the last five to ten years this has become normal practice in medicine. Those who have been into a hospital for an operation during that time might have been shocked when they were told the side-effects of a particular operation that they were about to have. If a procedure or treatment is about to be carried out, then the patient is told what might happen, good and bad. If the procedure is life-threatening or very necessary, then the patient knows what to expect if anything adverse happens and is not surprised or confused if it does. If that procedure might be avoided or changed to another procedure then that is something that can be discussed between the doctor and the patient after the patient has become knowledgeable about what is to be done. When the patient signs the consent form, then that is called 'informed consent'.

This principle should apply to all other types of therapies and treatments. Especially where the treatments are not regulated and there is nowhere to go if something goes wrong. People need to understand what they are choosing to have done. This is true in the field of cellulite treatments.

In talking to friends and family about cellulite, they all have their interpretation of what it is, what it is caused by, and what the treatments are. They have conflicting information. Some say that coffee and cigarettes contribute to cellulite. Others say it is stress or an outlet for illness deeper in the body. Even after reading up on the subject they are still confused about such matters as what detoxification is and so on.

Beat Cellulite Forever is all true. It is backed up by scientific research. It cannot be disputed.

There will be no need for confusion.

There are no vague statements.

If I do not know or cannot find the answer, I say so.

If it is true, I say so.

Dr James Fleming
Lancashire, England

◆

PART ONE

Cellulite and the Treatments Available

◆

CHAPTER ONE

What is Cellulite?

Definition

'CELLULITE' IS A POPULAR description used to describe the dimpled 'cottage cheese' or 'orange peel' skin, usually found on the thighs and buttocks of women. It is not a medical term and cannot be found in any medical textbook.

Ways of finding cellulite in a medical textbook would be to look up terms such as:

- hypo-lipodystrophy

- adiposis oedematosa

- dermo-panniculosis deformans

- status protrusis cutis.

Cellulite is a colloquial term used to describe the appearance of something. The terms above are different ways to describe the kind of tissue that cellulite is thought to be.

Types of cellulite

There are two main types of cellulite:

○ dermo-panniculosis deformans, which is full-blown cellulite, visible on relaxed skin with the naked eye; and

○ status protrusis cutis, which is cellulite that is only visible when the skin is pinched together between the fingers.

Its effects on women

It is a condition affecting 85 per cent of women who have gone through puberty and over 95 per cent of women over 30. Males are rarely affected.

Most women will agree that it looks unsightly, especially if it is extensive. Even exercise fanatics and female athletes can be riddled with cellulite. There seems to be nothing that they can do. There are few places to find information on the treatment of cellulite, particularly if you want to be sure that the information is accurate.

These are some of the reasons that women spend a lot of money each year on proposed treatments for cellulite. These treatments are often not regulated by the same bodies that regulate the use of conventional medicine. If something goes wrong there can be little recompense in these instances. It is an agreement between the women and the person providing the treatment.

Many thousands of beauty salons provide some treatment or other for cellulite. There is a small amount of treatment available from the world of conventional medicine, mostly constituting diet, exercise and surgery. Other areas to find treatments for cellulite are in the world of complementary medicine.

The internet is another source of treatments for cellulite.

There are thousands of websites, about 10,000 as a rough estimate, trying to sell a cure for cellulite. There are probably about 200 books on the shelves that mention the treatment of cellulite in some form. The books that tackle solely the subject of cellulite number about 20. Most of them agree with each other in a lot of respects.

What this book offers

This book will provide unique information on all the treatments for cellulite, the evidence or lack of evidence as to whether they work or not and a treatment plan based on all the cellulite remedies that are supported by concrete evidence to show that they are effective.

The standards that I use to determine whether a cellulite treatment works or not are:

1. clinical trials

2. logic

3. the experience of patients.

Clinical trials

In conventional medicine nothing is allowed to be used unless it has been proven to work by clinical trials. A clinical trial is research carried out under the most rigorous conditions. The results of these, usually undertaken by trained medical professionals, are often published in medical journals. If a doctor or another health-care worker knowingly submits an article to a medical journal that provides falsified results then he or she is immediately suspended from duty.

A full inquiry will then be started. This is because another health-care worker might read the article and change the way he or she treats someone as a result of this new research. Research in medical journals is taken very seriously and is seen to be the truth.

Logic

There are some treatments that I have come across that are not supported by clinical trials but that would logically work for the treatment of cellulite. For example, certain types of massage would logically reduce the appearance of cellulite because they improve the drainage in that area. They have been shown to improve the drainage by clinical trials but there has been no direct research involving that type of massage and the treatment of cellulite. This type of treatment is included among the treatments that work for cellulite. In time it is hoped that these treatments could undergo clinical trials. Until then it is enough to say that they will probably work.

The experience of patients

There are some treatments that have not been formally proven to work but that some patients have found very effective. Until the time when these treatments undergo formal clinical trials, if many women are happy that their cellulite is being reduced, then it is only fair that these treatments are included among the list of those that probably work. An example of this is 'body wrapping'. There has been no formal research on this subject but I have spoken to various people who swear that it works and some even claim that inches are lost from their thighs during a course of treatment. It would be unfair to the people involved in the treatments and those manufacturing the treatments to ignore such results.

The causes of cellulite

If the causes of cellulite are identified the best treatments can be selected from among the hundreds of available treatments on offer.

This is an extremely important part of the book. If you understand the causes and the structure of cellulite then you can take part in the logical analysis and appraisal of treatments for it. For example, if a treatment for cellulite proposes to rid you of edible toxins, thereby reducing the appearance of cellulite, you will learn later in the book that there is no way that this can work. There are no toxins in cellulite coming from what you eat if it is looked at from a biochemical point of view. Such a treatment plan might appear to work because a toxin-free diet is unavoidably a diet with fewer calories. You will become thinner and the cellulite will reduce in appearance. It is not the lack of toxins that is helping the cellulite, but the reduction in calories that you are eating. The facts are there for anyone to look at.

Structural causes of cellulite

First we can look at the structural causes of cellulite. A study in the US in 1998[1] showed that the fat tissue in cellulite was irregular in structure. Instead of the fat layer being smooth as it should be, and as it usually is in men, there are lumpy pockets of fat causing the skin above to be puckered and give the appearance of cellulite.

In this same study, and in one other,[2] no significant differences were noted between cellulite and normal fat. The parameters looked at included blood flow through the cellulite and through normal fat, and they suggested that the tissue separating the skin from the fat underneath is weaker if there is cellulite present.

The difference in the arrangement of the structure of the fat layer between males and females is largely due to the presence of septa (dividing tissue) in females that sequester the fat into pockets.[3] It is possible that these septa are the source of a low-grade inflammation that results in mild weakening of the overlying skin. This is only a theory though, and is not proven.

In both men and women the fat is separated into tiny boxes made up of collagen. Thousands of these tiny boxes make up a piece of fat tissue. In women the collagen is weaker so the boxes do not stand as squarely. This leads to the fat bulging and puckering, causing the appearance of cellulite.

Why fat structure differs between men and women

The structure of cellulite is hormonally rather than genetically controlled. Over two decades ago it was found that men affected with cellulite had a female tissue structure under their skin.[4] This research also found that the affected men did not produce enough male hormones such as testosterone. So, the presence of male hormones, not the lack of female hormones, such as oestrogen, stops cellulite forming. This means that the reason women get cellulite is because they do not produce male hormones.

Paradoxically, oestrogen can produce water retention, which has been cited as an important cause of cellulite.[5] The increased number of women taking the oral contraceptive pill, which is a synthetic oestrogen, has been suggested as an important factor in the prevalence of cellulite.

Different distribution of fat between men and women

In abdominal fat cells testosterone induces destruction of fat. This is why men can find it more difficult to put weight on than women.

In the thigh and bottom, oestrogen and progesterone enhance fat deposition. This is why women put weight on in those areas and men do not.[6]

Chemical causes of cellulite

There is another difference between normal fat and cellulite. Recent research in the US has shown that the proteoglycan content of cellulite is different from that of ordinary skin.[7,8] Proteoglycans are water-attracting molecules. An increase in skin glycosaminoglycans (a proteoglycan) has been reported in cellulite affected areas. In comparison, non-cellulite affected areas show normal skin structure, reflecting even distribution of structural proteins and glycosaminoglycans.

The role of excess fluid and toxins in the formation of cellulite

Fluid circulation and retention in the tissues has been given serious consideration in the creation of cellulite.[9] This is the theory of accumulation of toxins and water in adipose tissue, which is not being drained properly by the lymphatic system.

Various researchers have reported limitations of fluid movement and lack of lymphatic drainage contributing to the condition.[10] It is possible that localised swelling of the tissue results from inflammation and in this way contributes to the appearance of cellulite at the skin surface.

As to toxins, I said earlier in the chapter that it is possible that the dividing septa in the cellulite tissue of women are the source of a low-grade inflammation that results in mild weakening of the overlying skin. I also said that there are no edible toxins in cellulite. That is, nothing we eat can be called a toxin in the context of cellulite. The only things that may be called toxins in cellulite are the products of low-grade inflammation associated with the dividing septa in the structure of the cellulite tissue.

If the lymph is moving sluggishly for any reason these 'toxins' build up and may be a factor in the formation of cellulite. Unlike the blood system, the lymphatic circulation has no pump and is dependent upon muscular contractions to move it around the body. It is therefore suggested that a sedentary lifestyle causes poor lymphatic circulation, accumulation of toxins and water, and cellulite formation.

There are a few problems with this theory:

o It is unclear what these 'toxins' are in relation to cellulite. They only exist in theory in that context.

o Why do fit people get cellulite? Their circulation is clearly not at fault.

o By exercising to increase lymph circulation, how do we know that it is not the exercise and loss of weight that is improving the cellulite, not just increased circulation?

o If this theory does have anything to do with cellulite it can only be one factor.

o We do know that water accumulation has a part to play in the formation of cellulite. If this is due to sluggish lymph then this theory may have some truth. We know that the water accumulates due to increased proteoglycans in the cellulite as a result of a deformed structure of the fat tissue that it is made of. Is this proteoglycan a toxin? If it is then no dietary change will stop this except one where there is weight loss, then fat loss and then a reduction in the cellulite mass.

○ If proteoglycan is considered a toxin then there is no way to ever get rid of it because it is part of the cell structure.

So, the role of toxins in the formation of cellulite is unclear but it is worth considering. Any attempt at defining detoxification is difficult because it seems to differ from person to person. Even so, any attempt at a lifestyle that is toxin-free, however you define it, is good. If this helps the cellulite, then marvellous. If it does not, it has not done you any harm.

Sedentary lifestyle

A sedentary lifestyle is one in which we do not move around enough. For those who work long hours at a desk job it can be difficult to get moving. This kind of lifestyle is undoubtedly a factor in the formation of fat. More often than not in women this fat has the appearance of cellulite.

By increasing the amount of activity you do you will burn more calories, tone muscles, increase the capacity of the heart and lungs, and feel better.

Poor diet

Diet is probably the most important factor in the treatment of cellulite, along with exercise, for the majority of people.

There are people who have eaten well for many years and have kept an optimum weight with regular exercise, but who are still plagued with cellulite. There are many treatments in this book that work for the treatment of cellulite. So, if your cellulite does not respond to diet and exercise, that is the time to resort to other treatments, but for the majority of women, diet and exercise will be enough to markedly reduce the appearance of cellulite.

There are weight-loss diets and cellulite-specific diets outlined in this book, based on dietary therapies that have been proven to have a beneficial effect on cellulite.

Water and cellulite

Water is said to help get rid of cellulite. Many of the treatments for cellulite are based on getting rid of water. This is part of the theory of flushing the system. It all goes back to those toxins that are always being mentioned but that no one can describe.

Drinking a lot of water certainly helps to maintain health, but to suggest that it gets rid of cellulite is not based on any evidence. Also, we know that cellulite tissue has more water in it than other types of fat. That is one of its defining features caused by an excess of proteoglycans in the tissue.

It is undoubtedly good to drink plenty of water, but it is necessary to concentrate on other things for the treatment of cellulite.

Cellulite as a new problem

It is commonly thought that cellulite is a new thing, a result of modern food, lifestyle and toxins. My research suggests that women must have had cellulite for all time. It is only recently that women have started to wear fewer clothes and so make the cellulite more noticeable. Oil paintings done around the time of the Renaissance show the lumpy skin of women then, just as it is possible to see it now. Cellulite is not a new problem; it is just something people are now more conscious of.

When will you see results?

This is probably what you are wondering as you sit reading this. If you follow the plan in this book then you should start seeing results within a month – if you are committed and strict with yourself that is. There are so many treatments for cellulite outlined in this book that there has to be a plan for everybody, even those of you with the most stubborn cellulite.

How to use this book

Beat Cellulite Forever is divided into six parts. Part 1 explains what cellulite is and why most women have it. Part 2 looks at the pills and potions available to treat cellulite and includes anti-oxidants, diuretics and laxatives, and hormones. Part 3 looks at creams and lotions and also explores the surgical options. Part 4 looks at massage and complementary therapies, including body wraps and aromatherapy. Part 5 examines lifestyle options for beating cellulite, including diets, exercise and detoxing. Finally, in Part 6, I provide you with my easy to follow plan for getting rid of cellulite.

PART TWO

◆

Pills and Potions

◆

CHAPTER TWO

Anti-oxidants

What are they? The science

CELLS ARE SUBJECT to constant stress by substances called reactive oxygen species (ROS, also called free radicals). This stress has been implicated as a factor in a variety of degenerative diseases and in the ageing process. ROS are capable of causing adverse modifications of fats, DNA and proteins.

This is the connection with cellulite. It is proposed that ROS cause damage to fat cells and this leads them to degenerate and develop the appearance of cellulite.

Cells also possess anti-oxidant defence systems whose role is to minimise the effects of ROS. As you get older these defence systems do not work as well, which is why as people age they begin to look older and their bodies do not work as well. ROS are involved in a wide variety of human diseases including cancer.

Anti-oxidants are sold as remedies for many different things. The following is a précis of all the anti-oxidants on the market that are sold as remedies for cellulite. Whether they work is not proven and probably never will be in the case of cellulite, because there are too many variables. In theory, though, they should contribute something towards the reduction of cellulite. Few of them will do any harm and will almost certainly do some good somewhere in the body.

Are they worth buying?

Probably. They are like calcium supplements for osteoporosis. There is no direct evidence to suggest that anti-oxidants work for cellulite but people are advised they may take them because they will not do any harm and they might be beneficial.

Below are listed some commonly available anti-oxidants, with their properties, any side-effects and recommended daily allowance (RDA) in the case of substances I consider to be beneficial.

Juniper berries (*Juniperus vulgaris*)

Juniper is an anti-oxidant.[1] Like all anti-oxidants for cellulite it is hoped that it can help reduce the damage done to the fat cells by ROS.

Juniper berry oil is also an anti-oxidant and can improve the circulation in the small tubes of the liver.[2] It is probable that it would do so in other small blood vessels of the body. That is logically one of the reasons for its use as an anti-cellulite treatment, but there is no proof of this. Another reason is that it can lower the blood glucose level, according to a study done on rats.[3] The way it does this is by increasing the rate at which the body absorbs glucose from the blood. So you would still absorb the glucose, only a bit faster than if you had not taken the juniper.

Juniper berry oil has some diuretic properties, and is also used for indigestion, flatulence, and diseases of the kidney and bladder. It also has an antiseptic action when used as an oil.

SIDE-EFFECTS

Because juniper contains vitamin K, it can lessen the effect of oral anti-coagulant therapy [4,5] such as warfarin. People taking warfarin should not take juniper.

Large doses may cause irritation to the bowel.

Use it? **Yes.** It has many beneficial effects and will probably help cellulite.

RDA 425 mg/day, in supplement form, or eat them whole

Kelp (Fucus vesiculosis) and bladderwrack

Kelp, along with many other types of seaweed, is an antioxidant.[6] It also increases the metabolism, theoretically increasing the speed at which fat is burned. I suspect, though, that the amount of kelp you would have to eat in order to increase the metabolism enough to decrease the amount of cellulite significantly would either make you sick or cause side-effects.

There is no direct evidence to say that this works as a cellulite treatment but there is a chance that it would encourage weight loss. This is if you are prepared to tolerate the threat of a side-effect causing thyroid problems.

SIDE-EFFECTS

Kelp contains iodine. It is documented that if you eat too much kelp you might overdose on iodine, causing thyroid problems, such as weight loss, sweating and possibly goitre. Manufacturers of kelp as a dietary supplement advise that this might happen.

Use it?   **No.** The iodine content is too high. It is OK for the occasional meal but for everyday use the risk of side-effects is too great.

Black and green teas

A number of teas on the market claim to reduce the appearance or the level of cellulite. Looking at the medical trials on offer, many studies have been done on the various effects of tea.

Cellulite is supposed to have something to do with a build-up of toxins and damage to the cells in the affected area. That is the basis for using teas as anti-cellulite products.

RESEARCH
If blood is analysed for total anti-oxidant activity in a group of tea drinkers, results can be obtained showing that consumption of a single dose of black or green tea induces a significant rise in plasma anti-oxidant activity.[7]

A rise in anti-oxidant activity is beneficial to anyone's health, but it has never been proven that tea would have an effect in combating cellulite. I suspect, though, that tea is worth drinking while on a cellulite-reducing diet, because it might help in conjunction with other cellulite treatments.

SIDE-EFFECTS
As with most things that we ingest there are potential side-effects. The formation of cellulite is supposed to have something to do with an unhealthy blood system. Iron is needed to form blood. Herb teas, as well as black tea, coffee

and cocoa can inhibit iron absorption.[8] In someone who is iron deficient or who has a low blood count for whatever reason, tea can make this even more of a problem.

Use it?   **Yes.** Use it for it's antioxidant activity.

Peppermint tea

The basis for using peppermint tea as a treatment for cellulite is that it can act as a stimulant and will therefore raise your metabolic rate. As with all weak stimulants, though, a great deal of it would have to be taken in order to lift the metabolism significantly enough to cause any weight loss.

Because peppermint tea has a relaxant effect on the bowel it may cause mild weight loss, perhaps some fat loss and, according to people who sell the tea as a treatment, might reduce cellulite. Peppermint, however, slows the bowel down, so it would in fact be more likely to cause weight stabilisation or gain if anything.

SIDE-EFFECTS
Peppermint is safe.[9]

Use it?   **Yes.** It won't help cellulite, but tastes nice.

Aniseed tea and camomile tea

There is no evidence for these two teas having any effect on cellulite even though they are being sold in that capacity.

Use it?   **No.** Although it will probably help cellulite in conjunction with other treatments.

Milk thistle root extract (*Silymarin*)

As an alternative medicine milk thistle root extract is most widely used as a remedy for liver disease.[10] There is a potential, but unproven, benefit for this based on the free radical scavenger or anti-oxidant principle. Because of this anti-oxidant activity milk thistle has been added to the list of treatments for cellulite. If cellulite was in part due to lack of anti-oxidant activity, which we believe it is, then this treatment might work. To what extent, though, is unknown.

RESEARCH
There is no evidence for the use of milk thistle root extract in the treatment of cellulite.

SIDE-EFFECTS
Because of its effect on liver enzymes, there is potential for *Silymarin* to impair liver metabolism of certain drugs that are taken concurrently.[11]

Use it? **No.** It is not specific enough for its use as a cellulite treatment.

Dandelion (flower formula)

This aids the assimilation of vitamin B12, potassium and amino acids (valine and glutamine). It also aids the metabolism in the body of meat, game, shellfish, coffee, alcohol, sugar and other prospective liver harmers.

There is no evidence to say whether the substance is safe or not, or whether it works or not.

Use it? **No.** There is no evidence for the use of dandelion as a cellulite treatment.

Grape seed bioflavonoids
(*Proanthocyanidins*)

Grape seed 'addresses circulation, cellulite, toxin accumulation, and healthy metabolic process', according to suppliers of the substance as a food supplement.

Grapes and their seeds are well known for their beneficial effects, ranging from their anti-oxidant activity to their use as a bulk-forming laxative.

Proanthocyanidins are naturally occurring anti-oxidants found in grape seeds and many other fruits.[12] It is this substance in the grape that is purported to have the effect of reducing the appearance of cellulite.

Research shows that grape seeds are much better as anti-oxidants than vitamins C and E. This is one way of determining their effectiveness. Their direct effect on cellulite is unknown.

There is no evidence to say whether the substance is safe or not, or whether it works or not.

Use it? **Yes.** The anti-oxidant activity of grape seeds seems very good.

RDA 100 mg/day, in supplement form, or eat them whole

Guarana seed (*Paullinia cupana*)

Guarana seed 'is a natural stimulant and tonic, is used as an anti-stress agent, increases energy, acts as a diuretic, is a revitaliser and sustains the immune system', according to suppliers of the substance as a food supplement.

The seeds contain guarinine, which is basically caffeine, and tannic acid among other things.

It can be made into a tonic, which has effects similar to a stimulant, or even an aphrodisiac. It is also used as a diet drink in South America but in Europe its main use is for headaches. Guarana can be used to alleviate the symptoms of stress or tiredness, or for the discomfort of menstruation.

The cellulite-relevant activity of guarana is due to two of its constituents, estragole and anethole.[13] Anethole is an anti-oxidant.[14] Presumably so is estragole but there has been no formal research on this substance.

It might also treat cellulite due to its effect as a strong diuretic (it is capable of increasing the urine output five-fold) and its stimulant activity, which would increase the metabolism and make it slightly easier to lose weight.

SIDE-EFFECTS
There has been no formal research on any of its side-effects.

It should not be used by people with heart conditions or problems with the blood vessels, because in these instances it may increase the blood pressure.

Use it? **No.** It has not been tested properly.

Co-enzyme Q-10

Co-enzyme Q10 (ubiquinone) is a naturally occurring substance that is used as an anti-oxidant.[15,16] This substance is isolated from tobacco plants.

SIDE-EFFECTS
There is no evidence to say whether the substance is safe or not.

Use it? **Yes.** It may work for cellulite, but it is also being used for its anti-oxidant benefits.

RDA 30–100 mg/day, in supplement form

Pepper extract (*Piper nigrum*)

Black pepper is used as a stimulant, particularly for constipation, where it can be used as part of an enema to stimulate the bowel. It aids digestion and will help flatulence and nausea. This is one of the reasons for its use as a cellulite treatment, even though there is no direct proof for its use in this context. If it makes the bowels work more effectively that might be seen to aid weight loss, which has a beneficial effect on cellulite.

RESEARCH

A study on mice suggested that *Piper nigrum* (black pepper) helps the liver detoxification system.[17] This is another one of the reasons for its use as a treatment for cellulite. Piperine, a constituent of black pepper, showed a lower effect than *Silymarin* on the liver detoxification system but it did have an effect none the less.[18] This is a very vague reason for its use as a treatment of cellulite.

If this effect on the liver detoxification system is an aid to the work of anti-oxidants, then in theory a beneficial effect on the appearance of cellulite is possible, though unproven as yet.

SIDE-EFFECTS

There is no direct evidence to say whether large doses of pepper are safe or not, or whether they work for the treatment of cellulite.

Use it? **Yes.** It may not do a lot for cellulite, but seems to have a lot of benefits.

RDA eaten on food

White pepper (*Piper album*)

White pepper is from the same plant as black pepper. It contains no piperine, but one teaspoonful taken several times a day can be used to overcome severe constipation.

SIDE-EFFECTS
There is no direct evidence to say whether large doses of pepper are safe or not, or whether they work for the treatment of cellulite.

Use it? **Yes.** It may not do a lot for cellulite, but seems to have a lot of benefits.

RDA eaten on food

Cinnamon root extract (*Cinnamanum verum*)

Cinnamon has an effect of combating bacteria.[19] Eugenol, a component of cinnamon, may have an anti-oxidant action, which is the basis for its use in the treatment of cellulite. Its action as a stimulant may also be considered as having an action on cellulite, although this would be small and is as yet unproven. In any other context than as an anti-oxidant vast quantities would need to be eaten in order to combat cellulite. As an anti-oxidant, its action against cellulite is similar and as directly unproven as with any other anti-oxidant.

Its action as a cellulite treatment is as yet only theory but the theory is reasonably good.

SIDE-EFFECTS
There is no evidence to say whether the substance is safe or not, or whether it works or not for cellulite. I suspect it

would not do any harm though, as we all eat and enjoy cinnamon.

Use it?   **Yes.** It probably will not do much for cellulite. It tastes nice though.

RDA eaten on food

Onion

Onion has been quoted as a treatment for cellulite. It is an anti-oxidant.

Onion can be used as an antiseptic or as a diuretic. The juice can be made into a syrup, which is good for coughs and colds.

In the context of cellulite it must also be its action as a diuretic that has made it into a treatment. This would make more urine be passed, which might dry up the skin and the tissues underneath it. You would have to eat a lot of onions every day for this to occur and as soon as you stopped the fluid would return to the external tissues that had been depleted.

SIDE-EFFECTS
None that I have found.

Use it?   **Yes.** The benefits are very real here.

RDA eaten whole

Cloves

Cloves are very stimulating. They can be used for nausea, to cause vomiting, for flatulence and for general disorders of the stomach.

They can enhance peristalsis, which is the normal action of the bowel to move digested matter along it. Cloves are a powerful antiseptic. Cloves also possess anti-oxidant properties.[20]

The cellulite-relevant activity of cloves is that they are anti-oxidants and that they act as a laxative as mentioned above. There is no way of knowing how many cloves would have to be eaten to have a beneficial effect on cellulite.

SIDE-EFFECTS
Bowel cramps.

Use it?   **Yes.** Cloves have more than one anti-cellulite property.

RDA eaten on food

Turmeric

A study on mice suggested that turmeric and capsicum extracts could act as anti-oxidants.[21,22] The basis of turmeric as a treatment for cellulite is that it is an anti-oxidant.

SIDE-EFFECTS
None that I have found.

Use it?   **No.** Not enough evidence.

RDA eaten on food

Garlic and ginger

Garlic and ginger have anti-oxidant properties, but are described in greater detail in Chapter 4 and 5 for their other more potent anti-cellulite properties.

SIDE-EFFECTS
See pages 46 and 50.

Use it? **Yes.** Both these substances have multiple anti-cellulite properties.

RDA 1000 mg/day, in supplement form, for garlic; 550 mg/day, in supplement form, for ginger, or eat them whole

---

Substances with a good chance of having a beneficial effect on cellulite from Chapter 2

• Juniper • Kelp

If anti-oxidants are beneficial towards cellulite, and it has not been proven whether they are or not, then every substance in this chapter has a good chance of reducing the effect of cellulite, particularly the following, which have a cellulite action other than their known anti-oxidant action:

• pepper • guarana • cinnamon • onion
• cloves • turmeric.

◆

CHAPTER THREE

Fat-reducing Substances

I T WILL BE USEFUL to start with some definitions:

- **Cholesterol** – this is a solidified bile substance. Cholesterol is important in giving rigidity to the structure of cells and it also serves as a building block for bile acids and naturally occurring steroid hormones produced by the body such as oestrogen.

  The undesirable effect of cholesterol is in its contribution to the build-up of material that occurs over time on the inside walls of major blood vessels. This is called atherosclerosis and can lead to strokes, heart attacks and clots in the legs.

  If the amount of low density cholesterols (see below) is kept to a minimum, this build-up is limited.

- **Low density (LDL) cholesterol** – the type of cholesterol that is considered to be bad.

- **High density cholesterol** – the type of cholesterol that is considered to be good.

- **Triglyceride** – a normal type of fat. Our levels of triglyceride should be kept lower.

- **Fatty acid** – a normal type of fat. Our levels of fatty acids should be kept lower.

- **Lipid** – another way of describing fat.

The substances listed below are sold as cellulite treatments on the basis that they can lower the level of fat in the blood.

Salmon oil

Salmon oil has been cited as a treatment for cellulite. It has to be eaten, apparently, to have the desired effect.

One study from nearly 20 years ago compared the effects of eating salmon oil as opposed to vegetable oils.[1] The lower blood lipid levels and lower incidence of heart diseases and diseases of the blood vessels in Eskimo peoples suggest that the types of fats present in their diet of seal and fish may cause this effect. During the study the salmon oil diet reduced blood cholesterol levels and triglyceride levels. Harmful LDL cholesterol levels were also lowered. HDL cholesterol levels did not change.

If it is true that cellulite is made of fat, then anything that reduces the level of fat in the body would logically lower the incidence of cholesterol in that person. If we also presume that poor circulation has a part to play in the formation of cellulite, then any reduction of the deposits that build up in the blood vessels would also decrease the amount of cellulite in the body. Salmon oil seems able to do both of these things.

SIDE-EFFECTS
None that I have found.

Use it? **Yes.** This substance has a very good chance of helping cellulite.

RDA 130 mg/day, in supplement form

Omega-3 fatty acids

These are claimed to 'help balance blood cholesterol and healthy circulation' by their suppliers.

As well as their beneficial effects on the heart and the blood vessels, these fatty acids have anti-inflammatory effects and may also be able to reduce the amount of build-up on the inside of blood vessels.[2]

Higher doses of omega-3 fatty acids can lower elevated serum fat levels by 30 per cent to 50 per cent, minimising the risk of both coronary heart disease and diseases of the blood vessels.[3]

This might suggest that these fatty acids will have a beneficial effect on the blood vessels in cellulite, improving the circulation there.

SIDE-EFFECTS
None that I have found.

Use it? **Yes.** The benefits for health and for cellulite seem very clear.

RDA added ingredients to certain foods, such as some margarines

Soya lecithin

Lecithin beneficially alters the plasma concentrations of fats. In addition, it has been shown to lower blood levels of cholesterol.[4] Whether this has a direct effect on cellulite is unproven.

These results do suggest, however, as with all the fat-lowering substances, that lecithin may help to reduce the level of cellulite. How much it reduces the level of cellulite is not known or studied, nor is the amount of lecithin that needs to be taken.

Whether or not it has a beneficial effect on cellulite does not detract from the fact that this substance is exciting in terms of health because of its ability to lower cholesterol by significant amounts. Over a long period of time this can only help a person to reduce the risk of coronary heart disease and other diseases of the blood vessels, especially in elderly people who are more prone to these diseases.

SIDE-EFFECTS
None that I have found.

Use it? **Yes.** Good benefits for health, in fact so good that even if cellulite is not helped that much, the other benefits are worth taking it for.

RDA 1200 mg/day, in supplement form

Chromium tripicolinate

Chromium tripicolinate is supposed to 'reduce appetite and cravings as well as regulate and reduce the amount of body fat you store', according to those selling it.

The use of chromium as a treatment for cellulite is loosely backed up by scientific research. It has been proven to reduce levels of total cholesterol and LDL cholesterol.[5] This may contribute to a reduction of the appearance of cellulite.

The HDL cholesterol level is also elevated slightly, which is beneficial.

There are eight other studies like this, all on farm animals. The study I have quoted is the only human study.

SIDE-EFFECTS

None that I could find. This is because chromium has not been very thoroughly studied yet. As a metal mineral though, there are almost undoubtedly going to be side-effects with anything but the smallest doses of this when it is used as a food supplement. These would probably be things such as headache, nausea, tiredness and blood disorders.

Use it? **No.** Not enough research, no evidence.

Red clover

It has been suggested that red clover has an effect on the blood lipid levels. This is the only basis I can find for its use in the treatment of cellulite. There is no direct evidence to support this though.

RESEARCH

Red clover does not significantly alter plasma lipids in women with moderately elevated plasma cholesterol levels.[6] This is the only relevant clinical trial. It suggests that perhaps clover does not have the professed action of lowering the blood lipid levels. Unfortunately, though, this study is not relevant enough to cellulite to start drawing concrete conclusions from it.

SIDE-EFFECTS
None that I could find.

Use it?   **No.** Not enough evidence.

Hawthorn

Hawthorn can be used as a diuretic and to decrease the blood level of fats.

Its action on lowering blood lipid levels is only scantily supported by research.

SIDE-EFFECTS
Hawthorn may interfere with digoxin or with digoxin monitoring.[7] Digoxin is a drug given mainly to elderly people for disorders of the rhythm of the heart. Anyone taking it should not take hawthorn at the same time. There are no other side-effects that I have found.

Use it?   **No.** Not enough evidence. Not enough research.

Substances with a good chance of having a beneficial effect on cellulite from Chapter 3

- Salmon oil ● Omega-3 fatty acids ● Lecithin

◆

CHAPTER FOUR

Circulation-improving Substances

THERE IS LITTLE DIRECT evidence that cellulite is due to poor circulation of the blood in the vascular system. There is evidence that it has something to do with sluggish flow of the lymphatic system and also that a sedentary lifestyle contributes to the existence of cellulite.

It is logical that improved circulation would have a beneficial effect on cellulite even though proof of that is awaited. I have already shown that trying to remove toxins from cellulite by bettering the circulation is folly because there are no toxins in cellulite. There is proof, though, that due to an increased proteoglycan content in cellulite (see Chapter 1) there is an increased amount of water present in the tissue. Trying to remove as much of this as possible by bettering the circulation would probably make cellulite look less swollen and bumpy.

Whether you try to improve the circulation in either the lymphatic system or in the vascular system makes no difference, because by following the plan in this book, both will be improved.

Circulation in cellulite

The blood vessels in cellulite are small. There are three things that affect the circulation in small blood vessels:

1. damage to the vessels

2. the action of the muscles surrounding these vessels

3. the pumping action of the heart.

If the blood vessels in cellulite are damaged this will affect the flow of blood through the tissue. What may damage them is a sedentary lifestyle, sitting down all day or standing up all day. The blood vessels in cellulite are too small to be affected by atherosclerosis, the deposits of fatty material on the inside of blood vessels impeding the flow of fluid through them. The bigger vessels supplying the cellulite tissue may be affected by atherosclerosis though.

The blood in the small vessels in the cellulite tissue is pushed along by the movement of surrounding muscles. They have no pumping action of their own, like the bigger arteries, because they have no muscles. If the muscles are used less, then the flow of fluid through the cellulite is decreased.

Lymph and lymphatic vessels

The same is true for lymphatic vessels as for blood vessels, in that a sedentary lifestyle will make the flow of lymph through them weaker.

Lymphatic vessels are structures that are similar to blood vessels. They carry lymph away from tissue back to the central parts of the body. Lymph is the fluid outside the blood vessels in a tissue, which contains all the nutrients for that tissue to live on. It also carries away the waste products of metabolism from that tissue. It is very easy to damage these lymphatic vessels by vigorous massage.

If the heart is not working properly, or if it is never exercised, the flow of fluid through all tissues, including cellulite, is never quite as good as in those who exercise or who have a strong heart.

Improving circulation may reduce the appearance of cellulite even though it has not yet been proven. However, the benefits of even mild exercise will outweigh any drugs taken to improve the circulation.

White willow bark (*Salix alba*)

White willow bark is a natural and milder form of aspirin.

One of the main effects of aspirin is its ability to 'thin' the blood. It is very good at this and as such is one of the main treatments given to people who have suffered a stroke or a heart attack to prevent a recurrence.

Cellulite is reputed to be linked to poor circulation. White willow bark would mildly improve the circulation by thinning the blood.

There is no research evidence for its use in the fight against cellulite, but in theory it sounds like it might have some effect.

SIDE-EFFECTS
The same as for aspirin but not as severe. Side-effects are generally mild and infrequent, but include a high incidence of irritation of the stomach and upper intestine. Bleeding from the inside wall of the stomach may occur. Also clotting may be worsened.

It should not be used by people on warfarin or with bleeding disorders.

Use it? **Yes.** There is a strong possibility that this will do something for cellulite.

RDA 400 mg/day (15 per cent salicin) in supplement form

Horse chestnut (*Aesculus hippocastanum*)

This substance is claimed to 'promote the flow of oxygenated blood to all parts of the body' according to one supplier.

RESEARCH

It has been well documented that horse chestnut seed extracts alleviate the symptoms and reduce the signs of chronic venous insufficiency.[1,2] This is a disease of the blood vessels where fluid tends to pool in the legs and the tissues there because it is not being adequately transported back to the torso. All of the symptoms investigated – pain, tiredness, tension and swelling in the leg, as well as itching, improved markedly or disappeared completely. The results of this study show that treatment with horse chestnut extract is economical.[3] If cellulite is due to poor blood flow, then this compound would probably help to diminish cellulite in some way by improving the blood flow.

One study examined the effect of caffeine, horse chestnut, ivy, algae, bladderwrack, plankton, butcherbroom and soy protein all applied as a cream over 30 days. There was a 2.8 mm average decrease in the fat under the skin seen on ultrasound. It went back to normal as soon as application of the cream was stopped.[4]

Use it? **Yes.**

RDA 300 mg/day, in supplement form

Caffeine

Caffeine increases the metabolism.[5] This may help the fight against fat but quite a lot of it would have to be taken over a prolonged period of time for it to have a noticeable effect on cellulite. Cellulite treatment companies are picking up on this and adding it to the list of cellulite treatments on their menu. One such drug on the market is called Leptin.

SIDE-EFFECTS
These include sleepless nights, tremors, headache and dizziness. Over-indulgence may lead to a state of anxiety.

Use it? **Maybe.** Too much caffeine has side-effects though, as we all know.

RDA in coffee

Ginkgo biloba

Ginkgo biloba 'helps support normal circulation', according to some suppliers.

RESEARCH
Research suggests that ginkgo biloba extract can be used for intermittent claudication, a disease of the circulation where the patient cannot walk very far due to pain caused by a decreased blood flow in the legs.[6] This means that it must have a beneficial effect on the circulation, which might improve the appearance of cellulite. There is also evidence to suggest that ginkgo biloba may have a role in treating tissue swelling and inflammation, and may also act as an anti-oxidant.[7]

Ginkgo has strong anti-oxidant properties, protecting both the central nervous system and the cardiovascular system from ageing. It is currently being studied as an aid for impotence caused by impaired blood flow. Ginkgo strengthens tissue by stabilising cell membranes (aiding in the treatment of bruising and bleeding) and has been shown to increase not only the rate of blood flow to the brain, but the transmission of information to the nerve cells, enhancing memory ability. Ginkgo can also be helpful against tinnitus and vertigo, where impaired blood circulation can cause dizziness or ringing in the ears. Ginkgo may well be an important key in slowing down the ageing process as well as reducing the rate of free radical damage which can develop into cancer.

SIDE-EFFECTS
Ginkgo biloba may alter bleeding time and should not be used with drugs that thin the blood, such as warfarin.

Use it?   **Yes.** The benefits of ginkgo seem endless.

RDA 120 mg/day, in supplement form

Siberian ginseng (*Panax*)

Siberian ginseng is supposed to be 'the strongest form of ginseng, helping to increase energy levels, metabolic rate, and circulation', according to a manufacturer.

Chinese, Korean, Siberian and American ginsengs are currently used to enhance physical performance.[8] Improvements in muscular strength and heart rate have been shown, among other things, by the results of controlled clinical trials. This is another one of those cellulite treatments used on the basis that they are supposed to increase blood flow.

It is logical to presume that an increase in energy may result in more activity, and that may lead to easier weight loss. This is the basis for its use as a cellulite treatment, along with the fact that it can reduce the level of blood sugar.

RESEARCH

Ginseng contains many constituents. Among these, ginseng saponins are proven to be the most active constituents.[9] Ginseng saponins have positive anti-cancer, anti-inflammatory and anti-diabetes effects.[10]

The properties of ginseng are believed to be due to its effects on the hypothalamus, the pituitary and the adrenal glands, resulting in elevated plasma levels of certain stimulatory hormones.[11]

SIDE-EFFECTS

Ginseng may alter bleeding time and should not be used concomitantly with warfarin. Additionally, ginseng may cause headache, tremors and manic episodes in patients treated with phenelzine sulphate. Ginseng should also not be used with oestrogens or steroids because of possible additive effects in that ginseng might add to the effect of another drug making that drug more potent.[12] That means it should not be used if you take the contraceptive pill. Ginseng may affect blood glucose levels and should not be used in patients with diabetes. Ginseng may interfere with digoxin, a drug which increases the strength of the pumping action of the heart but slows down the conduction through the heart for those people with disorders of the heart rhythm. It may also interfere with digoxin monitoring, where its level is checked with blood tests. Too much of the drug in the blood may be dangerous.

Also, increased blood pressure, diarrhoea, restlessness and vaginal bleeding may occur.

Use it? **Yes.** If none of the side-effects listed above are likely to affect you.

RDA 500 mg/day, in supplement form

Wild yam root powder (*garlic*)

Garlic is used as an antiseptic. It also has effects as a diuretic and as a stimulant. Garlic is used to help with asthma, breathing difficulties and most other disorders of the lungs. It can cause you to cough up phlegm. It has long been established that garlic has a beneficial effect on blood pressure and on the heart. This is the basis for its use as a cellulite treatment.

RESEARCH
There is no research to prove that garlic has a beneficial effect on cellulite. From the vast research that has been done on garlic, though, it seems that it has so many good effects on the health that it might as well be eaten in abundance on the off-chance that it will improve your cellulite!

SIDE-EFFECTS
None that I have found.

Use it? **Yes.** It tastes nice and has a lot of good effects plus no side-effects.

RDA 400 mg/day, in supplement form

Cayenne powder (*capsicum*)

Cayenne is a powerful stimulant to the bowel, so is most useful in people who have a lack of activity of the intestines and stomach.

Cayenne 'opens every tissue in the body to increase blood flow, helping with metabolism and energy levels', according to manufacturers who would like people to use it for cellulite.

I could find no direct evidence for the action of cayenne powder on cellulite, although it may be argued that its effect on bowel movement may help in weight loss.

SIDE-EFFECTS
Stomach ache, loose bowels.

Use it? **Not really.** You would have to eat such a lot of it and it is very strong.

Substances with a good chance of having a beneficial effect on cellulite from Chapter 4

- White willow
- Horse chestnut
- Caffeine
- Ginkgo biloba
- Ginseng
- Garlic

◆

CHAPTER FIVE

Diuretics, Laxatives and Bowel Relaxants

Diuretics

A DIURETIC IS A substance that causes increased urination. Examples of diuretic medicines are Frusemide, Spironalactone and Frumil.

They work by increasing the rate at which fluid is lost from the kidneys to the bladder, and are mainly used by people who retain fluid due to a malfunctioning heart. This is where the heart is not pumping as strongly as it should, allowing a build-up of fluid in the lungs and the legs. This condition is referred to as heart failure. It is more common in older people and a large proportion of the elderly take Frusemide.

Many people think that they are retaining fluid but diuretics are not the answer unless there is something wrong with your heart or your kidneys. A normal kidney can cope even if you drink 150 litres of water in a day. This is because working at its most efficient, the normal kidney produces 120 ml of fluid per minute.

Many people complain of fluid retention in the legs. If you are worried about this then it should be checked by a doctor so he can listen to your lungs and decide about the serious-ness of any fluid retention.

Side-effects of diuretics are that they can upset the levels of certain substances in the body, mainly potassium. They can also lower the blood pressure to an unsafe level if not used properly. The principle of using diuretics as a treatment for cellulite is not sound because of the reasons explained in this chapter.

Ginger

Also called snakeroot in some parts of the world. It is grown in North America.

It is a stimulant, an anti-stress agent, a diuretic and an anti-spasmodic for the bowel.

Ginger improves bowel activity. In the context of cellulite treatments it would act as a laxative, giving the impression that weight was being lost.[1] This would allow the patient to think that fat was being lost from the cellulite areas. The weight loss would be transient and would last for the time that the ginger was being taken. There is no way of knowing how much ginger needs to be taken in order to have an effect on cellulite. Also, diarrhoea for weeks in order to produce a beneficial effect on cellulite is not ideal.

A significant decrease in blood glucose and cholesterol levels was found in rats fed a combination of garlic and gin-ger.[2] This would probably be true for humans as well. If the serum levels of these two things were reduced, less fat would be laid down so cellulite may decrease. However, the fat has to go somewhere even if a substance is taken to reduce its level in the blood.

Ginger is also well known as a healing plant for motion sickness, for vomiting in pregnancy and for stimulation of digestion.[3]

Ginger is recommended as a treatment for cellulite because of its many effects, not for one effect in particular. It reduces the amount of water in the body, improves bowel activity, acts as a stimulant and reduces blood levels of glucose and cholesterol.

SIDE-EFFECTS
Ginger may alter bleeding time and should not be used concomitantly with warfarin.

Use it?   **Yes.** Its many benefits outweigh its mild action in reducing blood sugar.

RDA 500 mg/day, in supplement form

Liquorice root

Liquorice is a popular remedy for coughs and chest complaints, such as bronchitis, and is an ingredient in almost all popular cough medicines on account of its valuable soothing properties. It 'stimulates the metabolism, increases energy and helps to regulate fluid retention', according to people who produce it as a treatment for cellulite.

The ingestion of liquorice can sometimes cause sodium retention, potassium loss and suppression of one of the systems that regulates blood pressure. What this has to do with the treatment of cellulite I am not sure. If it makes one pass water then maybe this extra fluid loss might make the skin seem a little tighter, giving a transient improvement lasting a few hours in the appearance of cellulite. So what? Consume too much and you will end up in hospital. Consume too little and the effect if anything at all will be temporary and negligible. Who knows what is too much and too little though? I don't.

One study had to withdraw people from eating 100 g of liquorice per day because their potassium levels fell too low to be safe.[4]

SIDE-EFFECTS

Liquorice can cause alterations in the blood pressure and swelling of the tissues.[5]

Use it? **No.** The evidence is not convincing.

Rosehips

An old wives' tale tells that this substance is a diuretic. It has been claimed to be a treatment for cellulite. There is absolutely no evidence for this.

SIDE-EFFECTS

There is no evidence to suggest whether rosehips are safe or not.

Use it? **No.** No evidence.

Uva ursi (*Arctastaphylos uva ursi*) (*bearberry*)

A study conducted on mice showed that uva ursi has some anti-diabetic properties.[6] This means that it lowers the concentration of blood glucose.

Uva ursi has also been shown to be a diuretic.[7]

SIDE-EFFECTS
None that I have found.

Use it?   **No.** Its safety is not assured.

Laxatives

Types of laxative and their actions

There are so many different types of laxative that it is useful to classify them. Even though only a few are sold as cellulite treatments and their action may only be temporary, so many people take them that I am including this classification.

There are five types of laxative:

1. **Bulk-forming laxatives** – such as bran and Fybogel. These laxatives cause there to be more volume to the faeces, which stimulates the bowel to contract more. The bulk also physically gets it all moving.

2. **Stimulant laxatives** – such as senna, cascara, bisacodyl and co-danthramer. These increase the movements of the bowel.

3. **Faecal softeners** – such as arachis oil, which is used for enemas.

4. **Osmotic laxatives** – such as lactulose. These act by retaining fluid in the bowel. They are not absorbed. By retaining fluid they give the faeces more mass and fluidity.

5. **Bowel-cleansing solutions** – such as picolax. These are only used to clean the bowel before surgery and are only available in hospitals. They are very powerful and even when used under direction from a doctor must be done so under the strictest guidelines.

Senna leaves (*Cassia angustifola*)

Senna is a laxative. It is the main laxative used in hospitals. Laxatives cause transient weight loss and this is the basis for their use in the treatment of cellulite. Some may argue that it may help to cleanse the bowel of toxins, hence the whole body, which would also help in the fight against cellulite.

Faeces contain toxins, but these are being constantly passed out of the bowel. Once faeces are in the bowel they are not reabsorbed by the body.

There is a school of thought that over time the bowel builds up a clay-like material on its inside wall, made up of toxins. It does not. If you look at a bowel with a camera passed inside the anus, what you usually see is beautiful, clean pink tissue with no residue attached to the walls.

The conclusion from this is that all a laxative will do in the treatment of cellulite is give the illusion that you are losing weight faster than you actually are.

SIDE-EFFECTS
Abdominal cramp, decreased calcium levels and prolonged use can cause the bowel to cease working.

Use it?   **Yes,** as a laxative. It may help cellulite temporarily.

RDA two tablets, at night, as required

Cascara sagrada bark

This is sold as a laxative with similar effects to senna.[8] Cascara is a powerful intestinal stimulant.

SIDE-EFFECTS
Abdominal cramp, decreased calcium levels and prolonged use can cause the bowel to cease working.

Use it? **No.** It is not used as a laxative any more in medicine.

Buchu leaves (*Betulina bosma*)

Buchu has long been known in Cape Colony as a stimulant tonic and remedy for stomach troubles, where it is infused in brandy and known as buchu brandy.

These leaves are sold as a cellulite treatment, but there is no evidence for their use in this capacity. I could find out very little about them. They are therefore potentially very dangerous because no one except the manufacturer knows about their safety and side-effects.

SIDE-EFFECTS
Unknown.

Use it? **No.** No way of knowing whether they are safe or not.

Bowel relaxants

Lavender

Lavender (*Lavandula angustifolia*) is used in aromatherapy as a holistic relaxant and is said to have calming, anti-flatulant and anti-colic properties.

Lavender has a relaxant activity on the bowel.[9] The mode of action of lavender oil resembles that of geranium and peppermint oils. The reason it is used as a cellulite drug is either because it has a calming effect and stress is supposed to have something to do with cellulite, or because its effects on the bowel have been wrongly assessed, as with the peppermint oil.

SIDE-EFFECTS
None that I could find.

Use it? It sounds quite harmless, but will not help cellulite.

Substances with a good chance of having a beneficial effect on cellulite from Chapter 5

- Ginger - Senna

CHAPTER SIX

Hormones and Cell Stabilisers

Hormones

A HORMONE IS ANY substance secreted by a gland, such as the thyroid gland, which produces the hormone thyroxine. Hormones act on cells or organs away from the gland to alter metabolism or growth.

Human Growth Hormone

Human growth hormone (HGH) increases the strength of collagen in the skin among a thousand other things. It also causes weight loss and decreases the amount of cellulite.

It is used in the treatment of growth hormone deficiency in children of short stature and for long-term kidney insufficiency. It can also be used for adult human growth hormone deficiency.

The safety of HGH as an anti-oxidant or as a treatment for ageing has not been substantiated by controlled clinical trials.[1] Human growth hormone is a very powerful hormone and its use as a treatment for something as benign as cellulite seems ludicrous.

Taking HGH does result in a reduction of weight gain in obese animals. It degrades fat and prevents it from being formed to some extent.[2]

SIDE-EFFECTS

The marketing of HGH is huge, especially in the US. It is such a fundamental hormone that its effects are almost too wide to define. Its potential side-effects include:

> headache, visual problems, nausea and vomiting, fluid retention, increased pressure in the brain, decreased thyroid function, reactions at the injection site, joint pains.

Do not use in the following situations:

> diabetes, pituitary gland disease, raised pressure in the brain, breast feeding, pregnancy.

Even though it has been marketed for use as a cellulite treatment, I'm not going to define it here any more than I have done. This is because in order to start such a treatment I think it should be under strict supervision from a hospital. It should not be used without such supervision. I would not prescribe HGH for something like cellulite, even though it would undoubtedly work. It is the side-effects that I would be wary of.

Use it? **Absolutely not.** Far too many potential unwanted side-effects. Far too powerful a substance to be used just for cellulite.

Cell stabilisers

Evening primrose oil (*Gamma linoleic acid*)

Evening primrose oil can be used as a sedative, in gastro-intestinal disorders, asthma and whooping cough.

It has been used to help dyspepsia (indigestion), and in certain female complaints, such as pelvic fullness associated with period pains.

Evening primrose oil is very widely used by women who find it very beneficial for different reasons. With so many happy customers the substance cannot be ignored.

As a treatment for cellulite it is said to 'support normal blood flow and hormonal balance' by those selling it. Clinical research to support the role of evening primrose oil in the treatment of cellulite is scanty. It has been claimed to improve allergic asthma; however, the evidence in favour of a useful therapeutic effect in this instance is poor.

RESEARCH

The most relevant reference found is an article in a German medical journal called 'Effect of topically applied evening primrose oil on epidermal barrier function in atopic dermatitis as a function of vehicle'.[3]

This study established the effect on the skin in patients with a condition called atopic dermatitis of evening primrose oil applied in a cream. Evening primrose oil had a stabilising effect on the stratum corneum barrier. This is the layer of the skin that makes it waterproof. This was apparent only with the water-in-oil emulsion of evening primrose oil. How it is applied to the skin is therefore an extremely important factor in the efficacy of evening primrose oil.

All we can guess from this study in relation to cellulite is that evening primrose oil stabilises one layer of the skin. Whether this reduces the appearance of cellulite or not is for the individual to decide.

SIDE-EFFECTS
Nausea, indigestion, headache, rash, itching, abdominal pain.

Evening primrose oil (and borage) should not be used with anti-convulsants because they may lower the seizure threshold. This means that they may make the epilepsy drugs work less effectively.

Use it? **Yes.** It may not work for cellulite but has many benefits.

RDA 500–1000 mg/day, in supplement form

Betaine HCL

Suppliers say 'it is a digestive enzyme. It speeds up the breakdown of foods. A more efficient digestive system increases the body's ability to use up body fat.'

Almost all cells are able to maintain normal cell volume without a disadvantageous response by the components that make up the cell. Betaine is one of the compounds that a cell accumulates in order to maintain a normal and stable cell size.[4]

Presumably if a cellulite cell is supposed to be deformed, producing the lumpy appearance on the skin, then stabilising the cells in that area will reduce the appearance of cellulite. From the available evidence though I do not think that conclusion can be drawn. Cellulite is lumpy because the pockets that contain lots of fat cells are weak. There is no evidence that there is anything wrong with the structure of any of the cells. The weakness is in the collagen that holds the normal fat cells in place. There is also no evidence that betaine has any effect on cellulite.

SIDE-EFFECTS
None are researched.

Use it? **No.** There is no proof for its use in cellulite.

PART THREE

Creams, Lotions

and Surgery

◆

CHAPTER SEVEN

Creams and Lotions

JUST AS WITH OTHER body creams, there are respectable names, well-known brands, expensive and cheap cellulite creams. For the treatment of cellulite, it is very important to look at the ingredients, more so than with a lot of beauty products.

Another factor in choosing a cream for cellulite is to look at its safety. Many manufacturers claim the creams have to penetrate the skin in order to have their effect. It is one thing to put any kind of moisturiser on the face, but it is another entirely to allow something that is potentially harmful to penetrate the skin and to enter the body.

> **Warning:** Not all cellulite creams are regulated by the same advisory boards that control production of most drugs and creams. Deciding on their safety may be up to the individual buying them.

The marketing of cellulite creams

A woman will buy a cellulite cream because she does not like her cellulite and because the media tells her that she should not like her cellulite.

For many of the creams available, the purchaser thinks that it probably will not work but it might, and it is worth giving it a try. This is important. The fact that cellulite creams are often not under the control of the advisory bodies that mainstream products are, means that it is up to you to ensure you are not buying anything unsafe.

If it seems a safe product and is supported by an extensive information leaflet then it is probably worth trying. Such information is often absent, however. This is when the cellulite treatment in question starts to look dubious in terms of safety and in terms of the effect it may have. Most of the available information can be found in this book, however. And the golden rule is, if in doubt, don't buy it. It is your body.

How to decide the safety of a cellulite cream or lotion

Any cream endorsed by a magazine that you trust is likely to be safe. Any major women's magazine is liable for the information that is in it, in spite of disclaimers like 'The magazine is in no way responsible for the safety of this product.' By the time a product for cellulite has made it into a women's magazine with a good reputation, it has already been used by a lot of people so should be safe.

A celebrity may use the product that you want to buy. If this is the case, find out how long the product has been on the market. If it is an appreciable length of time, over one year, then any major problems with its use should have emerged.

The cellulite product may be produced by a well-known brand name. This means it is probably safe. Such big companies are under the strictest safety guidelines for all their products. Unlike an internet vendor whose address you may not be able to find if the cellulite cream is being sold from someone's garage, a major company is liable for anything it sells. It will have a head office, shareholders and thousands of employees. If it becomes responsible for selling a product that is unsafe, it will lose business and its reputation.

How to choose cellulite creams

Rather than promoting individual brand names, Chapters 7, 8 and 9 on cellulite creams concentrate on the individual ingredients. You can look these up on the side of the jar in a shop or they can be searched for with ease on the internet.

Misconceptions

There is a school of thought that a cream might not get rid of the cellulite that is already there, but it may stop new cellulite appearing. If you can afford such a cream then it is worth a try, you think. This may be true, it may not. There is no evidence either way.

People do not really read labels. They believe that they know how the cream works. Just buy it and it does its job. Yet, for anything involving the body, reading the label is usually commonplace. Most people read labels for things they get from the family doctor. Products bought from a shop are not necessarily less potent.

Many cellulite creams are bought for their temporary effect, such as before an occasion where you will be wearing a short dress, particularly the skin tightening creams. This is probably a good idea as long as you remember that the effect is temporary and that the cellulite will return once you stop using the cream.

Some people think that a cream will dissolve the fat. None of them do. If this did happen it would be very dangerous. Where would the dissolved fat go? The only thing that can dissolve fat is your own body. Even so, when weight is lost, the fat is not dissolved, it is used for energy in a process where it is broken down chemically.

The cost

Cellulite creams are expensive, often twice or three times as much as a moisturiser. This is a good reason why many women might not use them, even if they wanted to. You may not be sure whether the cellulite cream works or not so your money may be wasted.

Exercise and a tightening moisturiser or cellulite cream are at the top of many women's lists for tackling cellulite when they set out to better its appearance. This is a reason why cellulite creams are such big business. As I have mentioned, it is the direct contact between the user's hand and their own cellulite that makes creams so attractive, among other things.

Do they work?

Yes, some of them.

There are many creams and lotions on the market for the treatment of cellulite.

Some of them tighten the skin overlying the cellulite. This gives a temporary improvement to the appearance of the cellulite. As soon as their use is stopped, however, the cellulite goes back to looking as it did before the cream was used. Such creams are good for the days running up to a beach holiday or an occasion where you would like to wear a short dress. For those creams that profess to tighten the skin on a temporary basis, the physical appearance of the skin after its use is the best way to judge.

Some creams are supposed to penetrate the skin and directly affect the cellulite, such as aminophylline cream (see Chapter 9).

The best way to judge whether they have a chance of working or not is by seeing what their molecular weight is. Only substances made up of particles of a specified molecular weight may penetrate the skin. The most important factor when discussing whether they work or not is whether they actually penetrate the skin and are absorbed. But note that if they are absorbed there is more chance that they will produce side-effects because they pass into the body.

The make-up of the skin

The outermost layer of the skin is called epithelial tissue. This tissue is avascular, meaning it has no blood supply. Blood is supplied from adjacent tissue. That means its nutrients filter across the tissue without going through blood vessels. This layer of tissue without blood supply is supposed to keep moisture in and unwanted substances out.

One layer of the epidermis (the outermost layer of the skin) is there as a barrier. This is called the stratum corneum. Most substances cannot penetrate the skin unless it is broken or unhealthy, because of the stratum corneum.

Molecules in cellulite creams

Some molecules can pass through this barrier layer, though, and if they are put into a cream they will have an effect. These molecules have to be very small.[1] In fact they have to be less than 500 Daltons in molecular weight. A Dalton is a very small unit of measurement used by chemists. Any substance bigger than 500 Daltons cannot physically pass through the skin to have its effect.

In Chapter 8, a third type of cellulite cream will be looked at. These are the creams that have a beneficial effect on circulation.

Substances with a good chance of having a beneficial effect on cellulite from Chapter 7

Creams containing molecules with a very small molecular weight, below 500 Daltons.

◆

CHAPTER EIGHT

Creams for Increased Circulation

THERE ARE ONLY A few creams that are sold for cellulite with the intention of increasing the circulation in cellulite.

Cellulite is a tissue like any other tissue. It is made up of fat cells encased in a structure made of collagen that keeps it together. The tissue has a blood supply made up of arteries that go into the tissue and veins that drain the tissue when the nutrients carried into it by the arteries have been drained away.

The tissue of cellulite also has a lymphatic system. The lymphatic system is a separate set of vessels running parallel to the veins that only contains lymph.

Definition of lymph

When blood passes into a tissue in blood vessels, it deposits its nutrients in a fluid that passes through the walls of the blood vessels. This fluid circulates around the tissue, deposits the nutrients, picks up the normal waste products of metabolism and is drained via lymph vessels, eventually back into the bloodstream. These products are not toxins.

Arteries, veins and cellulite

Creams that increase the circulation are supposed to work on the arteries and veins, not the lymphatic system. They should work on the circulation that we normally think of when someone says the word 'circulation'.

One common theory is that if the circulation in cellulite is increased, more water and toxins will be taken away from the cellulite and reduce its appearance.

This may be the case.

These creams are also said to improve the appearance and health of the overlying skin and make the whole structure of the cellulite more healthy.

This may also be the case.

There is no evidence to prove this in relation to cellulite. There is evidence, for example, that for people with leg ulcers, caused by poor circulation in the lower leg, rubbing aloe vera cream on the legs will help the circulation in the overlying skin and speed up the repair of the ulcer.

Most women who are concerned about cellulite do not have leg ulcers. By the time you get to the stage where you have leg ulcers, cellulite is the last thing on your mind. Even so, there are women with cellulite and unhealthy overlying skin. For these people, the use of a cream such as aloe vera will almost certainly improve the appearance of the part of their body that they are unhappy with.

So the creams improve the skin.

Whether they improve the circulation in the tissue that is cellulite is another matter. They can only do this if they penetrate the skin and have a direct effect on the cellulite, or if they have an effect on the whole body that improves the circulation everywhere and in so doing improves the circulation in the cellulite concurrently.

We do not want the effect of these creams to be on the whole body, we just want the areas with cellulite to have an increased circulation. The logic so far points to the effect of these creams being on the cellulite areas only, which is what we want.

I think it is reasonable to assume that if the skin overlying the cellulite has improved circulation as a result of using one of these creams, then there has to be some sort of improved circulation in the cellulite underneath. Also, all these creams seem safe and are being used widely for cellulite and for other problems.

Do they work?

They probably do. There is as yet no direct research evidence to support the use of a cream that improves the circulation on the cellulite tissue, but logic suggests that they are worth trying. Below are listed some substances that are said to increase circulation.

Aloe vera

Aloe vera, when swallowed, is capable of lowering blood sugar levels and of reducing the level of fat in the blood.[1] Applying it to the skin may have an effect on cellulite.

There is, as yet, no research to support an effect on cellulite, but when looked at with all the available evidence, logic suggests that it might help.

There is some evidence to support the use of aloe vera in people with stasis ulcers.[2] Stasis ulcers are the same as leg ulcers. This would suggest that it might improve the circulation. If cellulite has something to do with poor circulation, which it is thought it has, then this is a direction for the researchers to take when considering the effect of aloe vera on cellulite.

Otherwise, its effect on lowering the blood lipid level is probably going to mean that it might help cellulite if swallowed. As a cream it has not yet been proven to help cellulite. It probably will be though.

SIDE-EFFECTS
Aloe vera is very safe according to the research so far.

Use it? **Yes.** It seems safe, and will probably be proven to help cellulite soon.

Escin

Escin has been shown to be safe and effective for the treatment of chronic venous insufficiency (CVI).[3] This is a condition where the veins in the limbs collapse. This is also the full name for the disease that ends up causing leg ulcers. This might mean that it improves the circulation in the area in which it is used to some extent.

As a cream, escin seems quite hard to find. I could not find it apart from on the internet. As it has been part of a clinical trial though, it is something that I would be prepared to try for cellulite. There is a possibility that it might work for cellulite to some extent, but this is yet to be proven directly.

It is being used for venous problems in hospitals in various countries with some success.

SIDE-EFFECTS
None that I have found.

Use it?   **Yes.** Wait for more research if you are sceptical.

Echinacea

Echinacea is being sold as one of the cellulite treatments that is supposed to improve the circulation.

Echinacea increases bodily resistance to infection and is used for boils, septicaemia (blood poisoning), cancer, syphilis and other impurities of the blood, its action being antiseptic. It also has useful properties as a strong aphrodisiac. As an injection, its extract has been used for haemorrhoids.

RESEARCH
The main action of echinacea is directed towards the immune system.[4] There is no evidence for its use in anything resembling the treatment of cellulite.

SIDE-EFFECTS
If used beyond eight weeks, echinacea can cause liver poisoning and therefore should not be used with other known liver toxic drugs, such as anabolic steroids, amiodarone, methotrexate and ketoconazole.[5]

Use it?   **No.** No evidence for its use in cellulite.

Substances with a good chance of having a beneficial effect on cellulite from Chapter 8

- Aloe vera   - Escin

◆

CHAPTER NINE

Other Creams

Aminophylline cream

AMINOPHYLLINE CREAM seems to be big business. It is very easy to get hold of and many people are selling it as a treatment for cellulite. It is widely available over the internet and in some shops. It is a derivative of theophylline, which is used to relax certain types of muscle, for instance in the lungs, and to stimulate the heart. It also has some effect on making you pass water. It is very powerful and potent, normally only used in hospitals.

The basis of these creams is that they increase degradation or breaking down of fat cells. That it would cause spot fat degradation when used as a cream is a hypothesis.

More conventionally, the usual use for aminophylline is as a treatment for asthma, if other asthma drugs have not worked. When it is started in hospital for the first time the patient is monitored very closely because of the strength of the reaction that he or she might have to it.

A study in the *International Journal of Obesity* proved that aminophylline cream does not enter the bloodstream. How can it work then?

In one study of aminophylline cream, it was used with endermologie (see Chapter 11) for 12 weeks.[1] Endermologie is a machine-assisted massage system that allows positive pressure rolling, in conjunction with applied sucking pressure to the skin and fat tissues. The skin is rolled and then sucked back in an effort to smooth the contours of the cellulite. Its basis is to free the cellulite from any tethering underneath the fat and to smooth the lumpy fat pockets into a more uniform layer of fat.

In this study, body mass, thigh girth at two points and thigh fat depth measured by ultrasound were the parameters measured. No difference was found between those who had used the treatment and those who had not.

Even though there is a study to prove that the cream does not enter the bloodstream there are two more studies that report some reduction in the amount of cellulite after treatment with aminophylline cream.[2,3]

In one of these two studies the patients exercised and ate 800 calories per day for four weeks.

In the other just the cream was used and there was an average 8 mm decrease in the girth of the legs treated with the cream. Such a small loss could be accounted for by some transient skin-tightening effect of aminophylline cream that we do not even know about.

The message seems to be that there have to be more rigorous trials on this cream to investigate whether there is any potential at all for it to help the appearance of cellulite, while causing minimal side-effects.

SIDE-EFFECTS

No adverse effects have been noted yet with this cream except the odd rash. Absorption through the skin on areas of the body other than the thigh may be increased.

If someone finds a way for it to be better absorbed through

the skin and a level of aminophylline in the blood becomes apparent then the side-effects may be much greater. This is a very potent substance if it gets into the system.

There are no studies at all on the structure of amino-phylline cream, what it is and its potential general effect.

Use it? **Not yet.** Not enough evidence at the moment.

Topical retinoids

Topical retinoids are used on cellulite to tighten the over-lying skin. This reduces the appearance of cellulite for as long as the cream is applied.

These creams do work for the length of time that they are used. They cannot be used for a long time, though, without the fear of side-effects, such as the ones listed below. If used on the face they will cause tightening of the skin to an even greater degree, but the skin on the face is more sensitive and more prone to side-effects.

Topical retinoids can be found for sale in any shop that sells beauty products, even the supermarket. This suggests that any side-effects are minimal. If a major company is producing these, then they will have undergone rigorous testing. Also, supermarkets only take products from major companies subject to these tests. This is all in favour of the safety of topical retinoids.

They are useful for treating acne, but may cause some skin peeling and redness in that capacity.

SIDE-EFFECTS
Burning of the skin, stinging, itching, dry or peeling skin, increased sensitivity to sunlight, eye irritation, blistering or crusting of the skin. They should not be used in pregnancy or

when breastfeeding. This suggests that some component of the cream may be absorbed into the body.

Use it? **Yes.** Beware of potential side-effects though.

Cellulite gel

Cellulite gel makes the skin cold so is supposed to enable the tissue beneath to metabolise more quickly. An easier way of doing this would be to stand outside on a cold day in a pair of shorts.

In order to increase the metabolism by an amount that would begin to cause weight loss you have to be absolutely freezing for a good length of time, all over the body. The rate by which such a gel could increase the metabolism would be counteracted by eating half a biscuit more than usual in a day.

There is no evidence to say that this gel works.

SIDE-EFFECTS
None that I have found.

Use it? **No.**

Ivy cream

No references to this type of cream exist except those produced by people who try to sell it. Its mechanism of action and its efficacy are unclear.

SIDE-EFFECTS
None that I have found.

Use it? **No.** No evidence at all even to say what it is.

Snake root cream

There is no literature to say what this is or to prove that it works.

Use it? **No.**

Alpha-hydroxy acid creams

Alpha-hydroxy acid is another name for lactate. This is a derivative of lactic acid, which is formed when muscles are strenuously exercised. There is no evidence to say that it works for cellulite. Perhaps the manufacturers think that by putting lactate in the cellulite, it will con the body into thinking that it has just exercised so it will raise the metabolism in that area. There is no evidence to say that this is feasible, or that such an effect would occur, or that the constituents of the cream can even penetrate the skin to enter the cellulite tissue.

Perhaps this cream is just another skin tightener. Who knows. If the manufacturers will not even tell you what it is or how it works, why should you buy it?

SIDE-EFFECTS
None that I have found.

Use it? **No.** Absolutely not.

Substances with a good chance of having a beneficial effect on cellulite from Chapter 9

- Aminophylline cream   • Retinoid cream

◆

CHAPTER TEN

Surgery

THERE ARE VARIOUS TYPES OF SURGERY that are being used for sufferers of cellulite, from liposuction to microsurgery. From a doctor's point of view surgery is always the last resort. If the same outcome can be achieved without surgery, then surgery should be avoided.

Any anaesthetic that puts you to sleep carries a certain risk, although it is small. Complications of surgery are also possible. Certainly, for the treatment of cellulite, surgery should be the last resort. Some of the operations listed in this chapter are very interesting and produce fantastic results. There are reasons, though, why you should think very carefully before undergoing surgery:

• Why take the risk if you can get rid of the cellulite by another, safer method?

• Surgery is the most expensive of the cellulite treatments by far.

• Surgery for cellulite might not have the effect you were looking for. If this happens you will feel doubly cheated because of the risk you have undertaken and the money you have paid.

- During surgery requiring an anaesthetic you are unconscious and paralysed; your life is in someone else's hands.

Liposuction

Liposuction is remarkably effective for getting rid of fat. It is best used for localised fat over the hips, buttocks, thighs, knees and ankles, as it is very difficult to remove fat from these areas by dieting. The fat cells are permanently removed by this procedure so fat will not recur in that area.

It is not used in cases of obesity (where the body weight is 20 per cent more than the standard weight), because only a few kilos of fat can be removed at a time. If a lot more is removed there are physiological consequences that can make the patient very ill indeed. Patients who have loose skin need to know that they may have to have the skin tightened over the area where they have had liposuction in a separate procedure.

The number of people undergoing cosmetic surgery in the UK exceeded a million in 1998. The greatest number of procedures were performed on women aged 30 to 50, and the most common procedure was liposuction.

Liposuction involves inserting a tube into the layer of fat and sucking some of the fat out. It is not possible to get all the fat out, so if used for cellulite lumpy fat will still reside under the skin. If a smaller tube is used uneven fat removal can be avoided. If the fat is sucked out in a fan-shaped pattern this also reduces uneven fat.

After the operation the skin is flattened with a bandage for about a week so it heals in an even manner.

Studies indicate that this form of liposuction is of no use for cellulite.[1] The newer types of liposuction outlined below are said to work much better for cellulite.

SIDE-EFFECTS

The most frequent problem is an uneven removal of fat, which can be rectified some months after the operation with another procedure. There is usually a lot of bruising for some time afterwards.

Any operation carries a certain risk. The main risks of any operation are as follows:

1. **Infection** may occur after the procedure in the operated part, the adjacent tissue or in the lungs. (People are more prone to chest infections after surgery.) This is probably the most likely risk, but is still not that likely.

2. **Haemorrhage**, otherwise known as a bleed, after the operation or during it. This is not very common.

3. **A risk from the anaesthetic**, ranging from a drop in blood pressure during the operation to death during or after the procedure. This is even less common.

4. **Blood clot** after the procedure caused by immobility after the operation.

Use it?   **Yes,** if you want to. It is a well-recognised procedure.

Ultrasound-assisted liposuction

A new technique for the removal of fat by liposuction is called 'ultrasound-assisted liposuction'. Ultrasonic waves are passed through the fat before the liposuction is carried out. This prepares the fat by degrading it. The removal of fat is then more uniform because it is made more liquid and is easier to remove. This might have a more beneficial effect on cellulite, but still might leave the appearance of cellulite after the procedure.

It works in the following way. Ultrasound is capable of destroying living tissue in three ways:

1. It can heat the tissues up.

2. It can cause cavitation, which is where the ultrasound causes air bubbles (tiny) in tissue to grow. These wobble and break cell membranes in adjacent structures, such as cellulite.

3. Ultrasound destroys living tissue by direct mechanical action, which is how ultrasonic liposuction works.

Once the fat has been damaged and degraded by the ultrasound it is sucked out in the normal fashion. Using the ultrasound first leads to a better result in the end.[2,3]

There is less pain and discomfort when ultrasound is used first, and less swelling and bruising. No complications are reported with this technique.[4]

SIDE-EFFECTS
The same as for any kind of liposuction.

Use it?   Yes. The effects seem more promising than for normal liposuction.

Superficial liposuction

Superficial liposuction is said to be the most suitable form of liposuction in the treatment of cellulite. Superficial liposuction removes fat from just below the skin. After the procedure there is less chance that the appearance of cellulite will still be there. Normal liposuction involves the removal of fat from deep layers as well.

If the surgeon concentrates on the fat that is closer to the skin, there is more chance that the fat will be removed in an even manner, smoothing the appearance of the cellulite. If deep layers of fat are removed as well, there is more chance that some of the deep fat will be left, leaving the lumpy cellulite appearance that was there before liposuction.

Some people go for liposuction to have fat removed. Some go for liposuction to have the appearance of their cellulite improved. If the technique is being used for cellulite on a woman who is reasonably slim, there is no need to concentrate on the amount of fat that is removed. The only aim in such a procedure would be to better the appearance of cellulite.

The results of 2,500 patients having this cellulite treatment have been published in a medical journal and look very promising.[5]

SIDE-EFFECTS
The same as for any kind of liposuction.

Use it? **Yes.** The effects seem very promising.

Syringe liposculpture

Syringe liposculpture is removing fat from one place in the body and putting it in another place in the body. An example of this would be the removal of fat from the thigh to put in the breast.

For cellulite the treatment is called 'superficial syringe liposculpture'. This is a combination of syringe liposculpture and superficial liposuction. It breaks the fibrous tissue in the cellulite, which is another way of reducing its lumpy appearance. Again, results are very promising.[6]

SIDE-EFFECTS
The same as for any type of liposuction.

Use it? **Yes,** if you want to.

Tumescent liposuction

This is a technique of liposuction where the tissue is swollen first by the surgeons in an attempt to reduce the extensive bruising that can occur after the operation.

There are no studies yet on this type of liposuction.

SIDE-EFFECTS
The same as for any type of liposuction.

Use it? **Not yet.** Wait for the studies.

Keyhole surgery for obesity

Putting a band around the stomach to limit the intake of food through a keyhole in the abdomen is the surgical treatment of choice for obesity these days.[7] These bands are adjustable and also cause the least number of complications in patients.[8]

This treatment is for obesity, not specifically for cellulite.

SIDE-EFFECTS
The same as for any type of surgery, plus the risk of adhesions later in life. Adhesions are the abnormal joining of two

adjacent tissues or organs following surgery or inflammation. Symptoms range from abdominal discomfort to severe intractable pain, only relieved by further surgery.

Use it? **Yes,** if it is necessary.

Lower body lift with superficial fascial system suspension

This radical-sounding surgical technique might be recommended for someone with extensive cellulite, accompanied by fat pads on the hips and loose skin. It is called 'superficial fascial system suspension' or 'lower body lift.'

It involves lifting the skin of the whole lower body like a facelift in that region. It involves the skin of the flank, thigh and buttock. It is pulled up from the top of the hips to tighten the skin below it. Results can be excellent. The skin is pulled from the hips and lifted until the skin over the thighs and bottom has been tightened. Then it is fixed in that position. Before and after pictures from this procedure are fascinating – the fat and lumpy thighs and bottom are tightened into an appearance that is much smoother and slimmer.

If the skin is very lax after liposuction then a lower body lift can be performed. This seems like a big operation for the removal of the lumpy appearance of cellulite though.

SIDE-EFFECTS
These include infection, cysts, a prominent pubic bone and temporarily blocked lymph glands, as well as all the other potential side-effects of surgery.

Use it? **Maybe.** This is a major operation for a relatively minor problem. It works though.

Micro-surgery

Iontophoresis

This is a treatment device that uses direct electric current to introduce ions of soluble salts into body tissues for therapeutic or diagnostic purposes.

The only approved use for this at the present time is for diagnosing cystic fibrosis.

Even so, it is being used in some parts of the world as a cure for cellulite. The basis for its use in this manner is unclear.

There are no studies to prove its efficacy or its safety at the moment.

SIDE-EFFECTS
None that I could find.

Use it? **No.** No evidence.

Mesotherapy

This is injection of an enzyme into the cellulite to eliminate damaged connective tissue – the tissue that provides the supporting structure of the body around which other tissues are built. I could not find out what the enzyme is or how it eliminates damaged connective tissue.

This procedure is readily and widely available. There is undoubtedly damaged connective tissue in cellulite. If mesotherapy really does remove this and allows strong connective tissue to replace it, then it is a potential cure for cellulite. There need to be some rigorous clinical trials in the near future to give some figures on how well it works.

There are no studies to prove its efficacy or its safety. In theory it seems very promising. It should be carried out by a qualified doctor though, rather than in a beauty salon, because this is minor surgery.

SIDE-EFFECTS

None that I could find. I would presume that infection may ensue if the procedure is not carried out in a sterile manner.

Use it? **No.** Not enough research yet. Keep an eye on this one though.

Forms of surgery with a good chance of having a beneficial effect on cellulite from Chapter 10

● Superficial syringe liposculpture (works best)
● Ultrasound-assisted liposuction ● Superficial liposuction ● Stomach stapling ● Lower body lift surgery

◆

PART FOUR

Massage and Complementary Therapies

◆

CHAPTER ELEVEN

Massage

MANY PEOPLE THINK THAT massage may help the appearance of cellulite. This is part of the reason why they buy cellulite creams and lotions and massage them in. Some think that if the massage is too vigorous it will make the cellulite look worse. Others think of the fluid in the cellulite and believe that massage will help this.

After reading this chapter you will learn the truth about massage and its benefits because all of what I say is backed up by clinical research evidence.

Types of massage therapies

There are many types of massage therapy but each is based on a certain principle. All the available types of massage are covered below, apart from shiatsu, which is described in Chapter 12.

Hand massage includes:

○ Swedish massage

○ lymphatic drainage massage.

Machine-assisted massage includes:

○ endermologie

○ cellulite stick

○ hand-held electric massager

○ anti-cellulite deep massage appliance

○ deep heat, active air suction

○ hydro-massage

○ de-calcification

○ electric muscle stimulation.

Do they work?

Maybe. It is theoretically possible that some of the fat pockets may be ruptured by massage and result in reduction of the skin dimpling that causes the appearance of cellulite.

There are no studies to prove that machine massage helps cellulite, apart from the endermologie machine, which does seem to work, and apart from a suggestion, mentioned later in this chapter, that massage may reduce the fluid in cellulite.

Background

Massage is the basic form of all touch therapies. It is widely recognised to be beneficial to health. It is usually safe, very enjoyable and only involves the outer surfaces of the body.

It is used by healthy people who find it relaxing and invigorating. For the sick it is used to relieve pain and it can be beneficial simply to be touched by somebody else. It acts as a break in the role that the person plays throughout their illness as the receiver of sympathy and as the one who has a tendency to become depressed.

Anybody can benefit from massage if the technique is carried out by a qualified and sympathetic therapist. Even if the cellulite does not go away, you should leave the session feeling invigorated and relaxed. That has to be worth the money.

Swedish massage

Swedish massage is the technical name given to the type of massage where somebody uses their hands to rub the muscles and other parts of the body in an attempt to relax someone and make them feel good.

Swedish, or Western massage, based on body structure and muscles, tends to be used predominantly in sports centres and health clubs. Therapists use specific strokes to improve the circulation, tone muscles, ease joints and smooth out knots in connective tissue.

This type of massage has the same chance of reducing the appearance of cellulite as the unproven machine-assisted massagers described below. It is a lot more fun though. If it works, good. If it does not, it is still enjoyable.

There is no direct evidence to say that Swedish massage has any effect on cellulite, although it may well do. It is logical to assume that direct stimulation of an area of cellulite may improve the circulation in that area. It has not been proven that a bettering of the circulation in the cellulite improves its appearance but there is still a good chance that massage may help cellulite.

The effect may come from the fact that by having a massage, you are in a health club and are becoming aware of a part of your body that you are unhappy with. You may be more inclined to do a workout and to eat better. Over time, if you carry on this lifestyle, you will undoubtedly feel better, lose a bit of weight and the appearance of your cellulite will have improved. Even if this has nothing to do with the massage, if it helps with the lifestyle and is enjoyable then it must be worth doing.

SIDE-EFFECTS
None that I have found if it is done properly.

Use it? **Yes.** It's lots of fun and will probably help cellulite in some way.

Lymphatic drainage massage

Lymph is a collection of tissue fluid that is drained back into the veins via the lymphatic system. The lymphatic system is a separate set of vessels running parallel to the veins that only contains lymph.

When blood passes into a tissue in blood vessels, it deposits its nutrients in a fluid that passes through the walls of the blood vessels. This fluid circulates around the tissue, deposits the nutrients, picks up the waste and is drained via lymph vessels, eventually back into the bloodstream. By waste, I mean the normal waste products of metabolism. These are not toxins.

The only way that these waste products will not be removed is if the lymphatic system is blocked. This is a condition called lymphoedema. If this happens in one arm, for example, the arm will swell to twice or three times its normal size and you will be very unwell.

Faulty drainage of the lymphatic fluid is thought to be implicated as a cause of cellulite. Massage can help to drain away excess fluid from tissues.[1] Lymph can be counted as part of this excess fluid. It is probable that massage can help to relieve cellulite of some of its excess fluid.

After ten minutes of forceful massage, a study showed that damage of the local lymphatic system was present. The fluid in swollen tissue caused by excessive lymph can be removed by high pressure massage. Due to the high pressue applied, cracks develop in the lymphatic vessel walls and the fluid drains from the tissue through these.

Vigorous massage in swelling of the tissue due to excessive lymph also produces loosening of the tissue under the skin, and release of lipid droplets that enter the lymphatic vessels. By this mechanism, massage helps reduce the amount of fat cells in a leg that is swollen due to excessive lymph.

These findings suggest that massage may help to reduce the amount of fat in tissue, perhaps in cellulitic tissue. They do not suggest how much fat may be removed and they do suggest that vigorous massage of whatever kind damages the lymphatic vessels.

Another study gives the impression that manual massage drains lymph from tissues.[2]

SIDE-EFFECTS
Bruising, soreness and the probability of only a temporary effect.

Use it? **Yes,** if the masseuse is qualified. It will probably help cellulite.

Endermologie

Endermologie is a machine-assisted massage system that allows positive pressure rolling, in conjunction with applied negative pressure to the skin and subcutaneous tissues. The skin is rolled and then sucked back in an effort to smooth the contours of the cellulite. Its basis is to free the cellulite from any tethering underneath the fat and to smooth the lumpy fat pockets into a more uniform layer of fat.

Endermologie was originally developed in the late 1970s in France to soften scars.

Patients treated with the machine show improvement in body contour and skin texture. Since its introduction, endermologie machines have been used in many countries around the world in an effort to smooth the appearance of fat.

The results of one very relevant study showed that out of 85 patients, 46 patients completed 7 sessions of endermologie and demonstrated an average reduction in body circumference of 1.34 cm Thirty-nine patients who completed 14 sessions of endermologie showed an average reduction in body circumference of 1.83 cm. A decrease in average body circumference was seen regardless of loss or gain in patients' weight in most cases.[3]

One study demonstrated a 1.86 mm decrease in skin thickness after 12 treatments of endermologie.[4]

The company that pioneered endermologie is always careful to state that the product does not remove cellulite but reduces its appearance.

There are many other types of machine-assisted massage for the treatment of cellulite, which seem to be derived from the original endermologie machine. One is a great big, beaded, body-rolling machine. To quote the manufacturer, it is supposed to: 'stimulate the blood flow in the capillaries, speed up the removal of waste material in the intercellular spaces, aid the removal of excess fluid in the tissues, decrease water retention, speed up the process of tissue healing and repair, encourage the renewal of collagen, delay the signs of ageing, tighten loose skin and muscles, enhance bowel activity and stimulate the lymphatic system and therefore the immune system'!

SIDE-EFFECTS
None that I have found.

Use it?   **Definitely.** This is one of the top five proven methods to help cellulite.

Cellulite stick

This is one of my favourites. It is a large stick that you massage yourself with. I have visions of women beating themselves religiously with this stick in order to reduce their cellulite. It might work if it is done properly.

The problem, however, is that if a masseuse has to be trained for some time in order to do a good job, then how can someone who is untrained massage themselves with a stick? If the manufacturers think this is possible then they are cheapening the people who are trained in cellulite massage by saying that no training is necessary.

SIDE-EFFECTS
Aching arms from self-massage, bruising if done too vigorously, no effect if not done vigorously enough. These side-effects are merely my presumptions.

Use it?   **Yes,** if you are a trained masseuse, no if you are not.

Hand-held electric massager

This is a small electric vibrating machine that is supposed to make self-massage easier. It is for use on cellulite. A bit of a gimmick? It seems too small to massage vigorously enough, because if you press it on the skin hard enough for an effect, the motors stop whirring.

SIDE-EFFECTS
Not for use in the bath!

Use it?   **No.** Not powerful enough.

Anti-cellulite deep massage appliance

This is another electric hand-held massager that is a bit more powerful and has a vacuum bit on it. Perhaps it is like a small endermologie machine.

SIDE-EFFECTS
None that I could find.

Use it?   **Maybe.** I do not know how effective they are.

Deep heat, active air suction

This electric hand-held machine heats the cellulite up to some extent and then vacuums the skin towards the machine in an attempt to smooth the fat out. It sounds very dubious to me.

It might work, it might not. There is no proof either way.

SIDE-EFFECTS
No one knows because no one has formally tested it.

Use it? **No.** No evidence for its safety.

Hydro-massage

This is a shower that is quite powerful. By pointing it at the cellulite it is supposed to make it look better. It is known that massage must be powerful enough to damage the lymphatic vessels for it to reduce the amount of fluid in tissue or to break down the fat pockets and cause the cellulite to have a smoother appearance. The water surely cannot be powerful enough to do this. If it was it would knock you over.

SIDE-EFFECTS
None. It is just like being in the shower.

Use it? **No.** It doesn't work.

De-calcification

Ultrasound is used on cellulite in an attempt to reduce the levels of calcium in it (de-calcification). Ultrasonic waves are passed over the cellulite, which can then be massaged by hand afterwards to help clear away the calcium deposits through the lymphatic system.

The only problem is, there is no calcium in cellulite.

Ultrasonic de-calcification is being used medically for reducing the levels of calcium deposits in people with heart valve problems and this is the only research ever done on ultrasound de-calcification.[5]

The only time there is calcium in fat tissue is in calciphy-laxis, a rare disease that usually occurs in association with kidney failure and has a poor outcome.[6] The dermis layer of the skin and the fat under the skin is calcified.

The fact that people profess cellulite to be calcified fat is ludicrous. They may think that the blood vessels supplying the cellulite are calcified and therefore not as good at getting blood to the tissue. If this was the case you would be either so old or so ill that cellulite would be the least of your worries.

SIDE-EFFECTS

None for ultrasound.

For the hand massage afterwards, it is the same as for massage, i.e. ranging from none to bruising and pain with vigorous massage.

Use it? **No, no, no.** There is no calcium in cellulite.

Electric muscle stimulation

Pads are placed on one or two sites on the body. These are connected to a machine that passes small electric currents through the pads to make the muscles contract and then relax. It is making the muscles work repetitively, like being in a gym, but on a much smaller scale.

This may be a simple and effective method to improve muscle building, leading to better muscle mass.[7]

This technique is being sold as a treatment for cellulite and for being overweight or having lax muscles. You can sit and watch television while the muscles that the pads have been put on are given a light workout.

There are no studies to say whether this increases fat loss or has an effect on the appearance of cellulite.

We also know that it is not proven to obtain spot fat reduction from exercising the muscles underneath the layer of fat that needs to be removed. All the studies suggest that muscles are fuelled by fat that enters the circulation from fat deposits all over the body and that fat does not come down from a particular fat pad into the muscle mass next to it. Programmes where a particular part of the body is exercised and compared to another body part find that the concept of spot fat reduction has no basis. Therefore, even if electric muscle stimulation is very effective for increasing the muscle mass, fat can only be removed effectively by reducing overall body weight.

It is accepted, though, that by tightening the muscles under the cellulite this might give it a smoother appearance.

CONTRA-INDICATIONS

Because of what is stated in this chapter about temporary damage to the small blood vessels that may occur with massage it is probably better to avoid having areas with varicose veins massaged. Other conditions where massage should be avoided are:

o inflammation of the veins (phlebitis) – massage will make the condition worse;

o severe back pain – there may be something sinister underlying the pain that needs to be treated by a doctor, also a badly trained masseuse may aggravate some conditions of the back;

o blood clots – massage may lead to more blood clots if you are prone to them or may break up a clot, sending pieces all around the body to cause a stroke;

o women in early pregnancy may be better advised to abstain from massage.

Use it? **Yes.** It will probably help the appearance of cellulite.

Therapies with a good chance of having a beneficial effect on cellulite from Chapter 11

- Endermologie • Lymphatic drainage massage
- Electric muscle stimulation

◆

CHAPTER TWELVE

About Complementary Therapies

MANY TYPES OF complementary therapies are now available in the Western world. Many of them are based on ancient principles that have endured through the ages. This chapter deals with those that are being used to treat cellulite.

Manipulating complementary therapies include:

○ shiatsu

○ reflexology.

Shiatsu and reflexology will be covered in this chapter. Therapies using pills and potions are dealt with in Chapter 13.

Complementary therapies that use pills or potions include:

○ phytotherapy

○ aromatherapy

○ homeopathy

○ Ayurvedic medicine

○ Chinese herbal medicine

○ flower remedies.

Shiatsu

The word shiatsu means 'finger massage'. Its roots are in traditional Chinese medicine.

It works on the principle that disease is caused by a disturbance in the flow of energy through the body: this energy can be either depleted or blocked or overactive.

However deep the problem, it manifests itself on the surface of the body, at points called *tsubos*, via tributaries from the main channel of each meridian. The body's vital energy *qi* circulates around the body via the meridians or energy lines.

A shiatsu specialist can access the meridian by applying pressure at these points (the same points as are used in acupuncture), using thumbs, fingers, elbows, knees and feet. It eases musculo-skeletal tension and relieves stress.

There is no direct proof that this technique has any effect on cellulite but it is being used as a treatment for it. There are a lot of people though who are very happy with their shiatsu therapist and continue to have treatments.

SIDE-EFFECTS
It is very safe. It should not be used by people with osteoporosis or women in the first three months of pregnancy.

Use it? **Yes.** It's very pleasant. I cannot say it will help cellulite though.

Reflexology

Reflexology, or reflex zone therapy as it is sometimes called, is a treatment in which the practitioner applies pressure to the feet or less commonly to the hands in order to assess the health of the patient and promote well-being.

Having your feet massaged is very calming.

The science

Practitioners believe that all the body's organs, systems and parts are reflected in the feet. The foot can be mapped out to a very complex degree with every tiny area of it representing some part of the body.

By massaging the relevant point, the therapist stimulates the corresponding organs in the body, releasing natural healing powers. This is the claim of reflexology.

Lying down for a session of reflexology, letting someone else take control with their full attention on you, is deeply relaxing and therapeutic.

Experienced reflexologists say they can detect an area of disease in the body by feeling the foot. Crystalline deposits are said to build up in an area of the foot if the corresponding part of the body is diseased, and these deposits can apparently be felt under the skin of the foot.

Breaking down the deposits with manual pressure is supposed to begin the healing process. Thereafter the offending organ has been stimulated to heal itself.

Its uses

Reflexology is said to be able to help poor circulation, constipation, skin disorders and much more. Poor circulation is the basis for its use in the treatment of cellulite. Previously in the book it has been mentioned that there is an element of poor circulation in the areas of cellulite. Reflexology claims to be able to make this improve.

RESEARCH

There has been a lot of reputable research carried out on reflexology. The results are promising for the art itself, but not necessarily for the treatment of cellulite.

Patients with breast and lung cancer experienced a significant decrease in anxiety when treated with reflexology.[1] One of the three pain measures in the study showed that patients with breast cancer experienced a significant decrease in pain.

Reflexology has been shown to decrease flow resistance of blood in the blood vessels of the kidney. This has caused an increase in renal blood flow.[2] This shows that the art does have an effect.

Some might say that increasing blood flow in the kidneys means that blood flow in the cellulite could also be increased by reflexology. There is no proof of this yet. There may be in the future when someone researches it.

Research against reflexology

In a study of reflexology to assess its accuracy three experienced reflexologists were sent to see some patients without being told what was wrong with them.[3] They had to diagnose only from the patients' feet, given a choice of six diseases to choose from, one of which was the correct answer. They then had to rate the probability that each of the six conditions was present.

The results did not suggest that reflexology techniques are a valid method of diagnosis.

While reading this research though, I did wonder how well doctors would do if we had to guess a patient's condition from merely examining them and not talking. Probably not very well at all with many conditions if we could not use our blood tests and X-rays either.

Other studies concentrate on all types of disease and the effects of reflexology. The results are often promising.

SIDE-EFFECTS
None that I could find.

Use it? **Yes.** It may not be proven to help cellulite but it has potential benefits.

Therapies with a good chance of having a beneficial effect on cellulite from Chapter 12

- Shiatsu
- Reflexology

◆

CHAPTER THIRTEEN

Complementary Therapies Using Pills or Potions

Phytotherapy

PHYTOPHERAPY, OR WESTERN HERBALISM as it is also known, is becoming increasingly popular.

Western herbalism can be used for almost anything, but is said to be particularly good for skin complaints, stress-related conditions and menstrual disorders. Herbal medicines are taken as tinctures or teas.

A considerable number of herbs and plants have been found to be beneficial to health. The following are a few examples, all of which are being used for cellulite:

○ *echinacea purpurea*, a flower, is used to strengthen the body's immune system

○ ginger helps nausea and may relieve colds and flu

○ ginkgo biloba, extracted from the leaves of the maidenhair tree, is an anti-oxidant, improves blood flow and acts as an anti-coagulant.

SIDE-EFFECTS

Western herbalism is very safe in general, but an excessive intake of any herb could be toxic.

Little is known about the interactions between herbal medicines and conventional medicines.

Use it? **Not for cellulite.** There is no supporting evidence.

Aromatherapy

Aromatherapy is a very popular complementary therapy, which is being used increasingly in health and beauty clinics and in gyms. It is used in some hospital settings to help alleviate sleep problems, pain and stress, with some success.

Aromatherapy is based on the healing properties of essential plant oils. These oils cause the plant that they are extracted from to have its particular smell.

Essential oils are extracted from the flowers, leaves, fruit, seeds and bark of certain plants by steam distillation. They have a very complex chemical structure and each of the 400 plant essences that exist are said to have different properties.

How they work

The oils, in order to have their effect, are put on to the skin and some believe that they are absorbed this way. They can be inhaled or used in a bath as well. Indeed, some believe that the main effects of the oils are conveyed predominantly via the sense of smell and not by their absorption through the skin. Nobody really knows.

The sense of smell is connected with strong emotions and mood control. Aromatherapy can stimulate the release of neuro-chemicals as well as hormones into the body.

Because of their tiny molecular structure essential oils can easily be absorbed through the skin into the bloodstream. This is proven. Minute molecules of essential oil carried into the bloodstream are believed to affect different organ functions. Again, though, nobody really knows.

Types of treatment

There are three types of aromatherapy:

1. **holistic aromatherapy**, which uses essential oils and massage

2. **clinical aromatherapy**, which combines aromatherapy with conventional medicine

3. **aesthetic aromatherapy**, which is used by beauty therapists to relax people.

Because it encourages relaxation, aromatherapy is said to be good for stress-related conditions. Digestive problems also are said to respond well. During the aromatherapy session the massage itself will relax you.

Aromatherapy oils for cellulite

The following are some of the essential oils that are used for cellulite. There is no research yet, to prove that they work but that does not mean to say that they do not:

○ cedarwood

○ fennel

o juniper

o orange

o patchouli

o rosemary.

SIDE-EFFECTS

Essential oils can be lethal. They should never be drunk and should never be put neat on to the skin. If you have high blood pressure, diabetes, epilepsy, skin problems or are taking homeopathic medicines, you should avoid certain oils, which any good therapist can discuss with you. Pregnant women should only see a qualified aromatherapist. Aromatherapy is unregulated. Anyone can set up as an aromatherapist. There is no definition of what an aromatherapy product is. It ranges from toiletries that contain 3 per cent aromatherapy oils to 100 per cent pure oil. All can be bought easily.

Essential oils are very powerful substances. Bottles of essential oils are on unrestricted sale in the UK and need carry no danger warning. It is difficult to get detailed instructions on the side of the tiny bottles, but they can be put in a box with instructions and warnings in them.

RESEARCH AND MORE SIDE-EFFECTS

There is no research to say that aromatherapy works for cellulite.

One review of aromatherapy states, 'Aromatherapy massage has a mild, temporary calming effect. Saying that aromatherapy is effective for any other indication is not supported by the findings of rigorous clinical trials.'[1]

Essential oils of 11 plants are powerful in their ability to cause epileptic seizures.[2] Nine of them are eucalyptus, hyssop, pennyroyal, sage, savin, tansy, thuja, turpentine and wormwood. The final two are fennel and rosemary, and they are used for cellulite. They are discussed in detail below.

Fennel, as used for cellulite treatment

Fennel is a common British plant that is grown as both a herb and a vegetable. It also grows freely and is found in ditches and by the sides of ponds, although like mushrooms some wild fennel and is not safe to be eaten.

The part used for its medicinal action in humans is actually the fruit. It is the root that is eaten, while the seeds and leaves are used as a seasoning.

The fruits have been used for chest complaints such as bronchitis, tuberculosis and asthma. They have also been used for dyspepsia, fever and stomach ulcers.

In overdoses the fruits produce vertigo and a state similar to drunkenness. Externally applied, the root has sometimes been used as a remedy in piles.

Rosemary, as used for cellulite treatment

Rosemary is used medicinally as a tonic and a stimulant. Oil of rosemary is an excellent cure for headache. It is also used as a hair lotion, for its odour and effect in stimulating the hair roots to renewed activity and preventing premature baldness.

Use it?   **Yes.** It is pleasant but aromatherapy for cellulite is not supported by any evidence.

Homeopathy

Homeopathy is a system of medicine in which the treatment of disease depends upon the administration of minute doses of drugs that would in larger doses produce symptoms of the disease being treated. It was originated by Samuel C. F. Hahnemann (1755–1843), a German physician.

In a sense homeopathy is like giving a vaccine. The principle of homeopathy is that by giving someone the mild effects of a disease that the person already has, the person will have that disease cancelled out somehow.

Critics say that the concentrations of homeopathic medicines are so dilute that there is no way they can have any effect, but there is a study that says homeopathy can still have an effect even when the quantities are too small to be detected.[3] This is because it may work at a level in the cell of a human, possibly an electro-magnetic effect, that is unbelievably sensitive to even a mild stimulus.

Certainly, some swear by homeopathic medicine. I think it sounds quite exciting.

RESEARCH
There is no proof that homeopathy has an effect on cellulite.

SIDE-EFFECTS
Very few are reported.

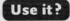 **Yes.** Not for cellulite but there are plans to introduce homeopathy into hospital for other problems.

Ayurvedic medicine

Ayurveda means 'the science of life'. It is designed to achieve a state of health through a blend of meditation, yoga, astrology, herbal medicine and dietary advice rather than alleviating or curing illness. It is practised widely in Sri Lanka and India.

Detoxification is one of the main principles underlying Ayurveda. Treatments used therefore include the application of warmth or oil massages to improve the circulation, medicinal remedies, yoga and dietary advice.

That is the basis of its use as a treatment for cellulite: circulatory improvement, exercise and a better diet. Certainly those three things would bring about an improvement in the appearance of cellulite. Whether increased circulation would have anything to do with it is not proven, but the diet and exercise component would help.

There is no research on Ayurveda as a treatment for cellulite. To become an Ayurvedic practitioner involves a five-year degree course in India. It has been practised for a long time and having a structured system to learn the practice at university of course makes it reputable. It can be practised alongside conventional medicine and as such I am certain there would be a lot of benefits from this system if it were more widely practised in the Western world.

SIDE-EFFECTS
None that I have found.

Use it? **Yes.** Its potential benefits seem huge.

Chinese herbal medicine

Chinese herbal medicine has been practised for over 5,000 years. It is the belief of Chinese herbalists that our health is determined by the state of our *qi* or vital energy and our *xue* (blood), which must flow freely for health.

Any imbalance in the components of *qi* (namely yin and yang) results in illness.

Herbs have one of five flavours (pungent, sour, sweet,

bitter or salty), five *qi* attributes (hot, cold, warm, cool or neutral) and four directions (ascending, floating, descending or sinking). The combination of these properties gives a herb a particular attribute or 'inclination'.

In Chinese medicine it is the manipulation of these inclinations, following the principle of opposites, that brings about balance.

RESEARCH
None that I could find. Certainly nothing related to cellulite.

SIDE-EFFECTS
There are very few side-effects that have been reported.

Use it? **Yes,** but properly with a trained practitioner. Might not help cellulite.

Flower remedies

Flower remedies are 'extracted' from the flowers of wild plants, bushes and trees by soaking the flower heads in spring water and boiling them. The principle of the therapy is that our emotions have a strong effect on our physical condition, and lifting our moods with flower remedies should improve our health.

Flower remedies are said to alleviate emotional and stress-related conditions. There is a school of thought that stress has something to do with cellulite. That is one of the reasons for the use of flower remedies in cellulite. Another is that if we improve our health we should reduce the amount of toxins in the body and of course cellulite is thought by some to be a symptom of sub-optimal health and a build-up of toxins (whatever they are).

Scientific analysis of flower remedies show that there is nothing in them apart from alcohol and spring water. No clinical trials exist to show that they work. They might do of course; we just lack any proof at the present time.

SIDE-EFFECTS
Flower remedies are completely harmless and can be taken by anyone.

Use it? **No.** Not enough evidence.

Problems with complementary medicine

Many people do not advise their doctor if they are using herbal medicines. There could be reactions with drugs that doctors may prescribe, so everything you take should be communicated to your doctor.[4]

Many people using complementary systems of medicine believe it is because of their lifestyle that they have their particular disease or problem. If the treatment does not work the patient ends up feeling guilty about having caused it or about not being able to get rid of it.

Occasionally people either do not visit the doctor at all or choose to discontinue conventional medical treatment. Complementary medicine can be extremely harmful if it is used as a substitute for proper diagnosis and treatment.

Eat sensibly and the body should remain healthy. Some therapists advocate the most ridiculous diets. For instance, people are encouraged to take vast quantities of dietary supplements, when some can be toxic in very small doses. Also, they cost a lot.

Therapies with a good chance of having a beneficial effect on cellulite from Chapter 13

- Phytotherapy
- Ayurvedic medicine

◆

CHAPTER FOURTEEN

Body Wraps, Sunbathing, Soaps, Sponges, Cloths, Rubs and Bath Liquids

SOAPS, SPONGES, CLOTHS, rubs, bath liquids, body wraps and sunbathing dry the skin and make it seem smoother temporarily. Drying the skin shrinks it slightly so may reduce the appearance of cellulite appreciably for a short period of time. A lot of these therapies do reduce the appearance of cellulite, but the effect is not long-lasting. This does not necessarily matter, though, if you are after a temporary effect for an evening out or for a beach holiday.

You cannot penetrate to the fat layer of cellulite by rubbing the skin. The only effect that it may be argued to have is one that is similar to a bad massage. It has been shown that in order for massage to affect cellulite it must be so violent that lymphatic vessels are damaged, allowing some of the fluid in cellulite to be pushed into them to drain away or for the fat pockets to be physically degraded. You cannot do that with a loofah without causing terrible damage to the overlying skin.

Body wraps

There are three types of body wraps outlined here:

○ normaform

○ rubber underpants

○ classic body wraps.

I do not see why all three body wraps should not work. I think they might have an effect on cellulite, although there is no research to substantiate this.

I spoke to the manager of a large beauty salon who assured me that the results with the body wraps are astonishing. She says that a client may lose 10 cm (4 in) in girth with one treatment. She also says that, with care, this loss in girth can be permanent. As she is my friend I have no reason not to believe her.

Normaform

This is a form of lymphatic drainage massage used in beauty salons. It involves the use of a pair of inflatable leggings. These are inflated very tightly to act as a kind of massage. The air pressure is designed to improve the natural circulation of the blood and lymph, and somehow get rid of excess water.

There is no direct evidence to say that this treatment works.

Use it? **Yes.** The results seem promising, if temporary.

Rubber underpants

This is another type of body wrap where women wear rubber underpants for about an hour to encourage the reduction of cellulite around their thighs. This has the same chance of working as any other body wrap. Even a beauty therapist who would admit that some of the treatments do not work so well would say that this and all other forms of body wrap show good results.

Use it? **Yes.** The results of this have not been formally quantified yet though.

Classic body wraps

This is where the affected areas of cellulite are wrapped in a substance like cling film for about an hour. This encourages sweating. Some therapists claim that it encourages a release of toxins through the skin, but in actual fact what is lost through the skin is only sweat, which is basically water, sodium and chloride, none of which are toxins.

Use it? **Yes.** This is a very popular treatment for cellulite.

Sunbathing

Sun exposure leads to structural damage in exposed skin. Glycosaminoglycans accumulate in sun-damaged skin.[1] This makes the skin look weathered eventually. The immediate effect of sun exposure is to dry the skin and colour it. This gives the illusion that the cellulite has improved. It might do for a few weeks. It may also tighten the skin and make it look smoother.

Who would deny that tanned skin looks better than pasty white? We all feel better when we get back from a holiday in the sun. Sunbathing undoubtedly improves the appearance of cellulite. As long as it is done safely, slowly and not too often, I cannot see a problem with it.

Sun safety

Sunshine contains ultraviolet radiation (UVA and UVB) that can cause skin damage, including sunburn and premature ageing of the skin, and this damage can lead to skin cancer.

Skin cancer is the most common cancer in the UK with the number of new cases diagnosed each year increasing. Each year there are more than 44,000 new cases of the most common type – non-melanoma skin cancer. In 1995 there were more than 5,000 cases of melanoma, which is the more serious and potentially fatal form of skin cancer.

The most important way to lower your risk of skin cancer is to avoid excessive exposure to the sun's UV radiation. There are some simple steps you can take to reduce your risk:

○ avoid the midday sun between 11 a.m. and 3 p.m.

○ take care not to burn in the sun – don't be fooled by a cool breeze or light cloud

○ cover up in the sun with loose cotton clothes, a wide-brimmed hat and sunglasses with UV protection

○ wear a sunscreen, of at least sun protection factor (SPF) 15 and a 4-star UVA rating, on areas of the skin which cannot be covered up

○ protect yourself while swimming – you can still burn underwater

○ children need extra protection. Keep babies younger than 12 months out of the sun completely

- look out for the solar UV index on TV weather forecasts at home and abroad

- there is no specific length of time to sunbathe for because it depends on temperature, humidity and where you are. The UV index on the TV should advise how long it will take to burn in the particular place you are holidaying in.

Finally, avoid using artificial tanning equipment.

SIDE-EFFECTS

Premature ageing, cancer of the skin, boredom while sunbathing.

Use it? **Maybe.** If you can cope with the potential risks.

Soaps

Soaps that are being used all over the world as a treatment for cellulite include lemongrass soap and oatmeal soap.

Lemongrass soap

No information can be found on this.

Use it? **No.**

Oatmeal soap

Oats act as a stimulant, increasing the excitability of the muscles.

Oat fibre, when eaten, is able to help lower cholesterol.[2] As a soap it has no effect on cellulite, because about 50 bars of it would have to be absorbed through the skin every day for it to work.

Use it?   **No.** No evidence to support its use as a treatment for cellulite.

Mineral waters

Whether these are drunk, bathed in or rubbed on, mineral waters are widely used for the treatment of cellulite. In fact, there is a large hotel in Switzerland dedicated to this very cause with its own mineral spring.

There is no formal research to say whether these waters have any effect on cellulite, but it would be a fun holiday.

It is not possible to find out what kind of minerals are in these waters and what their proposed effect is on any part of the body, never mind on cellulite.

SIDE-EFFECTS
Expensive.

Use it?   **Yes,** if you would enjoy such a treatment.

Alkaline mineral water springs

Washing your skin with alkaline water causes more water loss,[3] leading to drier skin. This would make the skin seem tighter for a short time, which might give the illusion of helping cellulite if the skin feels smoother.

SIDE-EFFECTS
None.

Use it? **Yes,** for the temporary effect.

Dead Sea mineral salts

Dead Sea salts contain magnesium bromide and magnesium chloride.[4] Their effect on cell growth is strong. They inhibit the growth of healthy skin. This may transiently improve the appearance of cellulite but there is no research to show this.

Dead Sea mineral salts can help the symptoms of rheumatoid arthritis after using them for only one month.[5]

Going to the Dead Sea also improves the symptoms of asthma.[6] If you can afford such a holiday you will come back tanned, invigorated and culturally more fulfilled. The cellulite would probably look better for a few weeks.

SIDE-EFFECTS
None that I have found.

Use it? **Yes.** For the temporary effect and for an interesting holiday.

Exfoliants

An exfoliant is anything that strips off the outer layer of an exposed surface on the body. The ones sold as treatments for cellulite are listed below:

○ loofah sponges

○ cactus fibres

○ wash cloths

○ horsehair mitts.

There is no research to show that exfoliants work and the principle behind their use is illogical. We know that cellulite is the fat under the skin. However much skin is removed by an exfoliant, it cannot affect the deeper tissue where cellulite is found.

Some therapists advocate vigorous skin-brushing four times a day to treat cellulite.

In Chapter 11 it was explained that research shows that in order for massage to make the appearance of cellulite better it had to damage the lymphatic vessels so their walls would break down and allow more fluid than usual to exit the cellulite tissue. Such massage would be so vigorous that it would cause bruising. To do this with a loofah brush, for example, would cause severe skin damage.

Another argument for using skin-brushing is that it is said to release toxins and improve circulation. Both of these have been examined earlier – toxins cannot be removed from cellulite and massage can usually only temporarily reduce cellulite. The theory that skin-brushing improves cellulite can only be because it is a form of massage.

There is no evidence to say that skin-brushing helps cellulite and with the reasons presented above I think anyone can see why.

Use it? **No.** There is no logic behind skin-brushing as a cellulite treatment.

Heating pads

These pads are put on areas with cellulite to heat the tissue up. The idea behind this is that the metabolic rate of the tissue increases so more fat is burned in that area. This might work if the pads were hot enough and if they were left on for hours and hours, but then the skin would be badly damaged. The same tissue can get hot just by sitting on it in front of the television in a warm room, so it seems illogical that heating a small area of tissue would get rid of fat.

Again, there is no research to prove that this treatment works.

Use it? No.

> **Products with a good chance of having a beneficial effect on cellulite from Chapter 14**
>
> ● Body wraps ● Sunbathing

◆

PART FIVE

A Healthier Lifestyle

CHAPTER FIFTEEN

Dieting for Life

IT'S WORTH REMEMBERING THAT dieting alone may not help cellulite as much as dieting combined with exercise.

Dieting for whatever reason has to be a lifestyle choice. It is tempting to lose weight for a few months and then to go back to eating as you did before the diet. Dieting is seen as a time of abstinence and suffering. You lose the required amount of weight and then go back to eating whatever you like in the hope of maintaining that new weight on the food that you ate and enjoyed before the diet was started.

It has been well documented that this type of abstinence diet does not work. However, a lifestyle change (for example, reducing the amount of sugar you eat) will be more effective in the long term. The weight may come off a bit more slowly, but it is more likely to stay off.

There are other factors involved in a lifestyle change. For instance, if you are one of those people who eats most in the quiet evenings, while sitting in front of the television, then habits need to be broken in order to lose weight. If you decide one day that you are not going to spend the evening eating in front of the television then you need to fill that time with something else, anything else. Otherwise you will eat because you associate that time and that activity with eating.

Celebrations can be difficult situations. It is possible to use food to celebrate everything. Going out for meals, entertaining and barbecues at home, Sunday roast and Christmas dinner are all examples of times when the temptation is to eat a lot because of the occasion. You feel a spoil-sport if you don't get involved in the festivities and the food.

You *can* make the choice to eat sensibly at all of these functions. After some time it will be as much a habit to eat well everywhere you go, as it is a habit now to think you will miss out if you do not have a huge ice-cream at the amusement park while you are in a situation to buy one.

It is useful also to think how much you would normally eat at a meal. If you have this in mind every day, then whatever you do you will stick to the healthy eating plan. It is a question of keeping mental notes of what you have eaten so far that day and how this compares to the ideal.

Here are some simple lifestyle changes you can make to start eating more healthily and to start getting rid of that cellulite.

○ If you are aiming to lose weight, try to lose 1 to 2 lb per week.

○ Think of a diet as being like buying a dog for Christmas. You are not going to get rid of it a few weeks later.

○ When you feel you want to eat but suspect that you are not actually hungry, think about the food you are about to eat and think about whether or not you are really hungry.

○ Eat simpler food. It will result in eating less because there is not the urge to try something new.

○ Get a regular eating pattern.

- Don't skip breakfast. This will probably lead to you eating 600 fewer calories per day.

- Don't skip meals. You will eat more in the long run.

- Don't fry.

- Grill, steam, bake.

- Drink something before a meal or have a light soup as a starter as this will prevent over-eating.

- If you are hungry, eat carbohydrates.

- If food is left over, get it out of sight.

- Eat slowly so the food can be tasted. It takes 15 minutes to feel full after you actually are full.

- Restrict eating to one room of the house.

- When you are hungry, eat. When you are full, stop.

- Restrict red meat to twice a week. Replace it with poultry, fish or non-meat meals.

- Eat fish at least twice a week.

- Eat lots of starchy food like brown rice, wholemeal pasta, bread, potatoes, beans and pulses.

- Eat at least ½ kilo (1 lb) of fresh fruit and vegetables per day, about eight portions a day.

- Use the guidelines listed on food packets to help you choose foods lower in fat, saturated fat and cholesterol.

- Use as little fats and oils as possible, but try not to cut them out altogether.

Dieting to lose weight

There are different ways of dieting to lose weight:

o eating less fat

o eating less

o food combining

o eating high protein, low carbohydrate diets

o and many more.

The basic idea behind all of these methods is that you cut out all the foods that make you fat and eat in a healthier manner. This invariably means eating less as well.

What to eat

Before we discuss specifics, here is a rundown of the nutritional needs for a person throughout the day.

Calories

Diets should include a minimum of 1200 calories per day, unless you are being supervised by a doctor. Going too low in calories can cause medical problems and unpleasant side-effects. Dizziness and lack of energy are the most common. For anyone with a busy life these symptoms are, of course, undesirable.

Also, if you eat less than 1200 calories per day your metabolism slows down because your body thinks you are starving. This is a natural mechanism to protect the body in times of famine and may actually prevent you from losing weight.

If you compare two people, one eating 1300 calories per day and one eating 800 or 900 calories per day, the following will happen:

1300 calories per day

Steady weight loss of ½–1.5 kilos (1–3 lb) per week

Easier to keep the weight off in the long term

Less temptation to binge eat or to have a quick energy fix like chocolate

Joy at the sense of achievement occurring with steady weight loss

A reduction in the amount of cellulite

800 or 900 calories per day

Headache

Tiredness

Lack of energy

Bad temper

Weight loss ½–1 kilo (1–2 lb) every two weeks

Much more difficult to keep the weight off long term

More temptation to binge eat and to have a quick energy fix like chocolate

A much slower, if any, reduction in the amount of cellulite

Protein

Diets should include about 55 g (8 oz) of protein per day. This is how much you need every day. Any more, and the source of protein, for example a piece of meat, may contain too many calories.

Carbohydrate

Diets should include a minimum of 150 g of carbohydrate daily (or about 600 calories). This is converted to simple sugars (the by-products of carbohydrate) which give you energy to move and to use your brain.

Remember, up to 40 per cent of your energy intake can be used by your brain.

Fat

Fat is a necessity in the diet. Fat is needed for many of the body's functions and without it the symptoms of deficiency will be experienced. These are:

o dry skin

o poor hair condition

o constipation.

Total fat intake per day should be around 53 g for someone on a 1600 calorie diet. However, no more than 30 per cent of the body's calorie intake should come from fat. The fat content of a food can be seen on the side of the packet. Some delicious low-fat, cellulite-busting recipes can be found in Chapter 16.

When dieting I think it is easier to eat simple foods because after a while the flavours start to be appreciated. If a person eats well on a low-fat diet for long enough, something very fatty will make them feel sick.

Mono-unsaturated fat

Mono-unsaturated fats are the healthy fats. They have been shown to lower LDL or the low density cholesterol, and increase HDL, or the high density cholesterol. As was explained in Chapter 3 LDL cholesterol levels are supposed to be low and HDL cholesterols are supposed to be high in a healthy person.

Roughage

In addition to watching the fat in your diet, increase the amount of fibre (roughage) you eat. Fibre is found particularly in cereals, fruit and vegetables. This will encourage the bowels to work properly.

Examples of food types and their place in the diet

The following table shows what form the various carbohydrates, proteins and fats might take, and shows how much of each should be eaten in comparison to the other.

Eat least	fats and oils	sugars and sweets	margarine and butter
Eat moderately	proteins	meat, fish, eggs, beans, pulses and nuts	milk, cheese and yoghurt
Eat most	carbohydrates	bread, cereals, grains, pasta and rice	potatoes
Drink lots	water		

Scientific research

Is misinformation being passed off as fact?

Because diet books and diet plans do not undergo scientific scrutiny as medical and health journals do, much of the 'science' reported is unproved and inaccurate.

Rate of weight loss

Losing more than ½–1 kilo (1–2 lb) a week usually signifies a loss not only of fat but also of muscle. If the diet is then stopped you then have less muscle and less chance of the next diet being successful. Also, in terms of cellulite you are trying to reduce its appearance. If the amount of muscle underneath is being decreased by a crash diet, the proportion of the overlying cellulite will remain the same so nothing will have been achieved with respect to cellulite loss.

Alcohol

In the Western world no chapter on diet would be complete without mentioning alcohol. Ideally it should not be drunk because of the 'empty' calories that it contains. The huge part that alcohol plays in everybody's lives, though, means that if it is stopped, it will not be for long. It is probably better, therefore, if you are aiming for a change in lifestyle, rather than a temporary diet, to plan for alcohol consumption.

The weekly recommended maximum for a man is 28 units (it used to be 21).

The weekly recommended maximum for a woman is 21 units (it used to be 14).

This is according to government health recommendations.

A unit of alcohol is:

o a glass of wine

o ½ pint beer or lager

o a normal measure of spirit.

A certain amount of alcohol can be good for you, however. By drinking two or three units of alcohol per day, you are actually at a lower risk of developing heart disease compared to drinking no alcohol.

◆

CHAPTER SIXTEEN

Cellulite-busting Recipes

THIS CHAPTER CONTAINS RECIPES featuring ingredients that act to reduce the appearance of cellulite.

Some of the ingredients are unusual. Putting them into recipes that taste good has taken longer to research than any other aspect of the book.

Here are the substances that I have included in the cellulite recipes, all of which have been shown to help in the treatment of cellulite.

Juniper	Caffeine	Ginger	Apple cider
Kelp	Fennel	Garlic	Onion
Salmon oil	Orange	Cayenne	Pepper
Lecithin	Rosemary	Cinnamon	Cloves

Next to each recipe is a text box with the names of the parts of the recipe that are there for reducing the appearance of cellulite. Combining these recipes with a healthy lifestyle and the kinds of low-fat foods mentioned in Chapter 15 will help to reduce the appearance of cellulite.

Wild mushroom and salmon salad

8 oz (225 g) can of salmon
12 juniper berries
1 glass of dry white wine
2 tbsp sesame oil
8 oz (225 g) wild mushrooms, sliced (or any type of mushroom)
2 garlic cloves, finely chopped
1 small onion, finely chopped
salt

METHOD
Drain the can of salmon and save the juice.

Put the salmon juice into a small pan with the juniper and wine. Bring to the boil and simmer for 3 minutes. Allow to cool.

Take the berries out of the stock and discard them. Fry the mushrooms, garlic and onion for 2–3 minutes in the oil.

Pour the stock into the pan with the mushrooms and cook for 1 minute. Add the salmon and the mushroom, garlic and onions.

Serve immediately.

4–6 servings. Per serving, 150 calories

CELLULITE SPECIFIC FOODS IN THIS RECIPE
• salmon • juniper • garlic • onion

Juniper pork

1 small onion, chopped
2 tbsp vegetable oil
1 tbsp dried red chillies,
  ground
12 juniper berries
3 cloves garlic, finely chopped
salt

1 oz (25 g) cooking chocolate,
  grated
³⁄4 pint (oo ml) of water
2 tbsp vinegar
3 oz (75 g) tomato paste
2 tbsp sugar
3 lb (1.5 kg) pork steak (loin)

METHOD

Preheat the oven to 150°C.

Cook the onion in oil until softened. Stir in the juniper berries, garlic and salt. Stir in the chocolate until melted. Cover and cook for 5 minutes, stirring occasionally. Stir in the chocolate until melted.

Pour the water, vinegar and tomato paste into a food processor. Add the onion mixture and sugar; cover and blend.

Place the pork in a shallow roasting pan, pour the sauce evenly over the pork.

Bake uncovered for 30 minutes. Turn the pork. Bake until done, about 30 minutes.

Note: the idea of mixing meat, chocolate and chillies comes from South America, around the time of the Aztecs. They also used to use the chocolate and chilli mixture with chicken and turkey.

6 servings. Per serving, 300 calories

CELLULITE SPECIFIC FOODS IN THIS RECIPE
• cloves • juniper • garlic • onion

Japanese salad

handful of sesame seeds
8 oz (225 g) thick egg noodles
1 lb (450 g) small prawns,
    cooked
8 spring onions, chopped
1 tbsp soy sauce

1 glass sake or white wine
2 tbsp grated fresh ginger
2 garlic cloves, finely chopped
1 tbsp seaweed, crumbled
1 tbsp sesame oil

METHOD

Toast the sesame seeds by dry frying until slightly brown, set
aside. In boiling water, cook the noodles until tender, about
10 minutes; drain, rinse and let dry. Transfer to a large bowl.
Add the prawns and spring onions; mix well. Blend in the
soy sauce, sake, sesame seeds, ginger, garlic, seaweed and the
oil. Cover and allow to cool .

Serve the noodles to make four servings

4 servings. Per serving, 250 calories

CELLULITE SPECIFIC FOODS IN THIS RECIPE
• seaweed • cloves • garlic • onion • ginger

Crab and seaweed salad with linguine

10 oz (275 g) fresh crab meat
salt and pepper
1 oz (25 g) Wakame seaweed
soy sauce
2 tbsp sesame oil
1 handful toasted sesame seeds
8 oz (225 g) linguine
3 tbsp peanut oil for frying

METHOD

In a bowl combine the crab meat, salt and pepper.

In a second bowl season the seaweed with soy sauce and 1 tbsp of sesame oil to taste. Dry fry the sesame seeds until they start to go brown. Sprinkle seaweed with sesame seeds.

Cook the linguine in salted water. Drain and add the other tablespoon of sesame oil. Mix the seaweed and crab. Serve over the linguine.

4 to 6 servings. Per serving, 250 calories

CELLULITE SPECIFIC FOODS IN THIS RECIPE
• pepper • seaweed

Lecithin bread made in a bread maker

Bread-making machines are readily available and very easy to use, and provide instructions on ingredients and use.

4 oz (125 g) lecithin granules
1 tbsp vitamin C powder
1 tbsp ginger, ground

METHOD
Mix together the ingredients above.

Add a measure of the ingredients that is equal to your yeast measurement, and add to the other dry ingredients needed to make the bread. Alternatively you could add 1½ teaspoonfuls of the lecithin per cup of flour. The lecithin and ginger is to add to the normal ingredients of the bread.

CELLULITE SPECIFIC FOODS IN THIS RECIPE
• lecithin • ginger

Fish pasta

1 lb (450 g) rigatoni pasta
1 tbsp olive oil
1 lb (450 g) cod fillet, cut into bite-size chunks
2 cloves garlic, finely chopped
1 tsp fennel seeds
1 red pepper, diced
1 can (28 oz/800 g) chopped tomatoes
2 tbsp fresh basil, chopped
salt and pepper to taste

METHOD

Cook the pasta in boiling water. While the pasta is cooking, heat the olive oil in a large saucepan. Add the cod, garlic, fennel seeds and red pepper, and cook for 8 to 10 minutes, until the cod is tender. Add the tomatoes. Cook for a further 8 to 10 minutes, until the sauce has thickened. Stir in the basil. Drain the pasta, transfer to a serving bowl, then pour the sauce over it. Season with salt and pepper.

4–6 servings. Per serving, 570 calories

CELLULITE SPECIFIC FOODS IN THIS RECIPE
• fennel • pepper

Orange chicken

4 oz (110 g) margarine
2 small cans concentrated frozen orange juice (6.7 oz, 190 g)
2 oz (50 g) breadcrumbs
½ tsp salt
½ tsp pepper
4 cloves garlic, finely chopped
1 tsp paprika
4 large skinless chicken breast fillets
4 oz (110 g) plain flour

METHOD
Preheat the oven to 150°C (300°F, gas mark 2)
Melt the margarine with orange juice in a frying pan. Put a small amount into a bowl to coat the chicken. Mix breadcrumbs with seasoning. Roll chicken in flour, then in orange and margarine mix, then in breadcrumbs. Transfer the chicken to a shallow baking tin. Pour the rest of the orange mix around the sides of the chicken. Bake for approximately 40 minutes.

4 servings. Per serving, 250 calories

CELLULITE SPECIFIC FOODS IN THIS RECIPE
• orange • pepper • garlic

Herb mix for dressings and dips

2 tbsp parsley flakes
6 tbsp mixed herbs (sage, thyme, marjoram, oregano and parsley)
1 tbsp sugar
1 tbsp fennel seeds, crushed
1 tbsp dry mustard
1½ tsp black pepper

METHOD
Place all the ingredients in a jar, cover tightly and shake well to mix. Store in a cool, dark, dry place.

One tablespoon of mix: calories 13, total fat 0, saturated fat 0.
Note: This low-sodium, low-fat mix can be stored for up to 6 weeks.

CELLULITE SPECIFIC FOODS IN THIS RECIPE
• fennel • pepper

Ginger-flavoured stir-fried chicken

4 chicken breasts, boneless and skinless
⅓ cup plain flour
1–2 tbsp oil
3 floz (100 ml) fruit juice (orange, apple, pineapple)
2 tbsp honey
2 tbsp soy sauce
½ tsp powdered ginger
½ tsp garlic, finely chopped
mixture of vegetables (mange-tout, broccoli etc)

METHOD
Cut chicken into 2-in pieces. Coat with flour and heat oil in a wok. Cook chicken pieces in hot oil for 2 minutes.

Meanwhile, mix together juice, honey, soy sauce, ginger and garlic. Pour mixture over chicken and cook 2 minutes more, until sauce thickens slightly. If sauce becomes too thick, add up to ¼ cup water.

Add mange-tout and cook and stir until vegetables are crisp-tender. Serve over white rice.

4–6 servings. Per serving, 300 calories

CELLULITE SPECIFIC FOODS IN THIS RECIPE
• orange • ginger • garlic

Herbal vinaigrette dressing

1 tbsp herb mix (see page 145)
3/4 cup (200 ml) water
2 1/2 tbsp white wine vinegar
1 tbsp olive oil
1 clove garlic, finely chopped

In a small bowl, whisk all the ingredients together. Taste and add ¼ to ½ tsp of the herb salad dressing mix if you want a stronger flavour. Let stand at room temperature at least 30 minutes before using, then whisk again.

One tablespoon of dressing: calories 25.
Note: This low-sodium, low-fat mix can be stored for up to 6 weeks. If you make salads often, double the quantities.

CELLULITE SPECIFIC FOODS IN THIS RECIPE
• fennel • pepper • garlic

Seafood seasoning mix

½ tsp salt
2 tsp dried red chilli flakes
1 tbsp finely ground black pepper
2 tsp paprika
1 tsp garlic powder
1 tsp dried basil
⅛ tsp dry hot mustard
1 tsp ground bay leaves
¼ tsp thyme
¼ tsp tarragon
½ tsp oregano
½ tsp rosemary
(use dried herbs)

METHOD
Mix all ingredients together well. Store in a tightly covered glass jar for use as needed. Excellent for seasoning all seafood. Use as you would any seasoning mix, and do not add extra salt to the dish.

About 4 calories per teaspoon

CELLULITE SPECIFIC FOODS IN THIS RECIPE
• pepper • onion • garlic • rosemary

Italian tomato sauce

3 tbsp olive oil
½ onion, finely chopped
1 clove garlic, minced
1 rib celery, diced
1 small red pepper, diced
28 oz (800 g) can crushed tomatoes
28 oz (800 g) can chopped tomatoes
6 oz (170 g) can tomato paste
herbs (preferably fresh, but dry will do) in amounts according
to your own taste: basil, sage, rosemary (crumbled), oregano,
thyme, marjoram, parsley, salt, dash crushed red pepper flakes
3 large courgettes, sliced medium-thin

METHOD

In olive oil, in a large soup pot, sauté onion, garlic, celery
and pepper until tender. Reduce heat; add all of the canned
tomato products. Stir well to combine. Add all of your sea-
sonings. Remember to adjust to your own taste. Stir well.
Add courgette slices and stir well. Bring to a gentle boil.

Reduce heat and simmer on a very low heat for about 2
hours, to blend the flavours. Be sure to stir every now and
then. May be easily reheated on stove top or in microwave.
Great as a vegetable dish, or on cooked spaghetti. Italian
bread is a complement to this dish.

4 servings. Per serving, 200 calories

CELLULITE SPECIFIC FOODS IN THIS RECIPE
• rosemary • pepper • garlic • onion

Baked seasoned salmon

1 level tsp salt
8 juniper berries
1 tbsp dried rosemary
pinch cayenne pepper
½ tsp ground ginger
½ tsp fennel seeds

½ tsp garlic salt
¼ tsp black pepper
2 salmon fillets (chilled)
2 tbsp olive oil
2 oz (50 g) samphire or
    asparagus

Method

First, make the seasoning:

Pound all the dry ingredients to a powder with a pestle and mortar, then distribute evenly over a plate.

Heat a non-stick frying pan and when it is hot dip both sides of the chilled fish fillets into the olive oil and then into the seasoning blend on both sides.

Fry until just starting to brown on both sides or until cooked through.

Serve on a bed of samphire (steamed without salt) with a wedge of lemon, and accompanied by some fresh bread.

Note: Samphire (Glasswort) is grown in Norfolk, UK between June and August.

2 servings. Per serving, 350 calories

CELLULITE SPECIFIC FOODS IN THIS RECIPE
• salmon • juniper • rosemary • ginger • pepper
• garlic • fennel • onion

Spicy fish curry

2 cardamom pods
8 juniper berries
1 tbsp coriander seeds
½ tbsp curry powder
a pinch of cayenne pepper
4 tbsp olive oil
1 tsp grated fresh root ginger
1 onion, chopped

4 cloves of garlic, finely
  chopped
1 bulb of fennel, chopped
1 oz (30 ml) coconut cream
½ pint (250 ml) water
juice of a large lime
4 salmon fillets
2 fresh rosemary sprigs

METHOD
Grind the whole spices in a mortar and pestle. Heat the oil in a wide frying pan and add the spices and curry powder.

Fry for about 3 minutes, then add the ginger, onion, garlic and fennel and cook until the onion and fennel has softened. Dilute the creamed coconut with ½ pint of water and add to the pan with the juice of a lime.

Place the salmon steaks in the sauce and continue to simmer for about 10 minutes or until the fish is just cooked through. Garnish with fresh rosemary sprigs.

Serve with fresh bread to mop up the juices.

4 servings. Per serving, 350 calories

CELLULITE SPECIFIC FOODS IN THIS RECIPE
• salmon • juniper • cayenne • ginger • fennel
• garlic • rosemary • orange • onion

Glazed carrots

20 oz (550 g) baby carrots
2 oz (50 g) brown sugar
2 tsp cornflour
1/4 tsp ground ginger
4 oz (110 ml) orange juice

METHOD
Cook the carrots. Cover to keep warm and set aside. Place the brown sugar, cornflour and ginger in a medium-sized saucepan, and stir to mix well. Slowly stir in the orange juice. Place the saucepan over medium heat, and cook, stirring constantly, until the mixture reaches a boil. Continue to cook, stirring constantly for about 1 minute, or until the mixture has thickened.

Add the carrots to the glaze, and stir to mix. Cook, stirring occasionally, for 1 or 2 minutes, or until the carrots are hot and well coated. Serve immediately.

4–6 servings. Per serving, 200 calories

CELLULITE SPECIFIC FOODS IN THIS RECIPE
• orange • ginger

Spicy fruit punch

2 cinnamon sticks, each 3 in long
½ tsp whole allspice
½ tsp nutmeg
12 whole cloves
4 pt (2 l) cranberry juice cocktail
4 oz (110 ml) maple syrup
2 tbsp fresh lemon juice
4 pt (2 l) apple cider
orange and lemon slices studded with whole cloves for garnishing

METHOD

Place the cinnamon, allspice, nutmeg and cloves on a small muslin square, bring the corners together and tie securely with kitchen string. (If you don't have muslin, add the spices to the juice and pour the mixture through a sieve before adding the cider.)

In a soup pot, mix together the cranberry juice, maple syrup and lemon juice. Add the spice bag and place over medium heat.

Bring to a boil, reduce the heat to medium-low, and simmer for 20 minutes to blend the flavours. Remove from the heat, cover and let steep for 15 minutes before adding the cider.

CELLULITE SPECIFIC FOODS IN THIS RECIPE
• cinnamon • cloves • apple cider • orange

Iced fruit salad

1 can (1 lb (450 g)) pineapple chunks, in natural juice
2 oz (50 g) sugar (or equivalent in artificial sweetner)
1 can (8 oz (225 g)) mandarin oranges, drained
1 can (8 oz (225 g)) apricot halves, drained
2 bananas, sliced

METHOD
Drain pineapple, reserving the liquid. Add water to the pineapple juice to equal 1 cup and add sugar, stirring until dissolved. Add all the ingredients to the juice. Cover and freeze for several hours or overnight. Let it sit at room temperature for about 30 to 45 minutes before serving.

4 servings. Per serving, 80 calories

CELLULITE SPECIFIC FOODS IN THIS RECIPE
• orange

Fruit in ginger sauce

½ pt (250 ml) vanilla low-fat yogurt
2 tbsp crystallised ginger, finely chopped
4 small navel oranges, peeled
8 ripe strawberries, hulled
2 medium bananas, peeled

METHOD
Place the yogurt in a small bowl. Add the ginger, and stir briskly for about 1 minute, or until the yogurt has a sauce-like consistency. Set aside. Cut each orange crosswise into 5 slices. Cut each strawberry lengthwise into 4 slices. Slice the bananas. Spoon ¼ cup of ginger sauce onto each of 4 plates, and spread the sauce over the plate. Arrange orange slices around the plate. Arrange the strawberry slices around the plate. Add banana slices and serve.

4 servings. Per serving, 80 calories

CELLULITE SPECIFIC FOODS IN THIS RECIPE
• orange • ginger

◆

CHAPTER SEVENTEEN

Exercise

IT IS A FACT THAT any exercise will help the appearance of cellulite wherever it is on the body, if that exercise is regular over a prolonged period of time.

Regular exercise helps to tone up the heart, lungs and muscles, as well as keeping bones strong to reduce the risk of osteoporosis in later life. It is important to start exercising gently, and then to build up gradually, otherwise you can put your body under excessive strain. If you are in any doubt about your fitness to exercise, have a chat with your doctor.

How to start

If you start to exercise too fast you will develop fatigue in the muscles over a week or two, this might make it difficult to climb the stairs or to do a full day's work. If you combine excessive exercise with an inadequate diet that leaves you nutritionally deficient you are likely to end up in bed feeling ill after a short period of time. Starting more slowly means that you can carry on exercising indefinitely.

To some extent, the type of exercise is less important than the fact that you actually do some. It is recommended that the ideal amount of exercise is 20 to 30 minutes, three to five times a week, and that you should exercise to a level that makes you a bit breathless. Whatever the exercise, if it is done to this timescale, the cellulite will start to reduce in appearance.

If you want to start checking your pulse rate during exercise, then aim for 65–70 per cent of your maximum heart rate (MHR) to start with. Your MHR is defined as 220 minus your age, so if you are 44, your MHR would be 176. Initially, you would aim to exercise to keep your exercise pulse rate to 75 per cent of MHR.

Exercise such as swimming, cycling or walking will help to improve your level of fitness. If you decide you want more and join a gym, then make sure you take expert advice with regard to types of equipment, and vary your exercise between muscle building and cardiovascular exercise.

Many people are overweight. A lot don't accept it: statements such as 'I've got big bones' or 'I've always been big' are just excuses, nothing more. A small proportion of people might have a slower metabolism or might be more predisposed to being overweight. If you are not happy with your weight or your cellulite then excuses do not matter. The fact is, that is the body you have and whatever needs to be done to make it the way you want, has to be done by you.

Body mass index (BMI)

A number of years ago a formula was devised by the US insurance industry, which linked weight to life expectancy. This is the result of dividing your weight (in kg) by the square of your height (in metres), and is known as the body mass index (BMI).

BMI is $\dfrac{\text{weight (in kg)}}{\text{height}^2 \text{ (in m)}}$ e.g. $\dfrac{100 \text{ kg}}{2 \text{ m}^2} = 25$

A normal BMI is between 20 and 25.

The following table shows the significance of different BMIs in adults:

BMI (Body mass index)	Health status
under 20	underweight
20–25	normal
25–30	overweight
30–35	obese
over 35	seriously obese

The principles of exercise

It is important to understand the principles of exercise. If you are trying to get rid of cellulite, a sensible, complete exercise programme is all that is needed to burn away some fat. This way you won't overdo it and you will have more chance of the exercise becoming a life decision rather than something that is done temporarily. The exercise should be enjoyable and lead to feeling better and more healthy, not something to be dreaded because it is so hard.

There are six parts to the principles of exercise:

1. enjoyment

2. flexibility

3. cardio-respiratory

4. strength

5. endurance

6. rest and recovery.

Enjoyment

There are ways to make sure that you enjoy exercise. Before you start any exercise you have to think about what you are about to do. Take away any of the worry or hassle associated with it before you start.

- **Consult your doctor.** If you have any medical problems at all, then see your family doctor before you do any exercise. Your doctor will advise you about anything you need to avoid or be careful with. If you get the OK from your doctor then you can stop worrying about whether it is going to be harmful to you.

- **Decide what exercise you are going to do.** Many people join a gym. This is the most sensible course of action, especially if it has been years since you have exercised. You can begin with a rounded programme tailored to your needs and as non-stressful as possible to the temporarily weak joints of your body.

- **Pick a gym near to your home.** Very near. That way you are more likely to go if it is only round the corner. Imagine it is the middle of winter. You are just home from work, and it is your gym night. The thought of a 45-minute drive to the gym is more than enough to make you think that for tonight you can avoid it. If you have any other plans for that evening, then you will start to resent the amount of time it takes for you to go to the gym.

- **Pick a gym with nice changing rooms.** I once attended a gym, briefly, and the only reason I stopped going was because the changing rooms were so cold, I could not face it any more.

- **Pick a gym offering exercise classes.** All you have to do is turn up. Once you are in the class there is no backing out. On those days when you lack motivation you will still get a good workout.

- **Pick a cheaper gym.** They can be just as good as a very expensive one and you will not end up resenting all the money you pay just for the privilege of a workout.

Flexibility

Being flexible decreases the chances of sustaining muscular injury. Flexibility exercises are those that gently stretch muscles and ligaments, before, during, after and in between workouts.

Cardio-respiratory

This refers to the capability or fitness level of your heart, blood vessels and lungs to transport oxygen to your tissues.

Aerobic exercise must be performed to increase the level of cardio-respiratory fitness. These are exercises that utilise oxygen during the activity, that put up your heart rate and make you breathe more deeply and more frequently. It is exercise that is performed continuously and is usually rhythmic and repetitive. Examples are walking, jogging, running, skipping, skiing, cycling, swimming and rowing.

For fat burning, more intense exercise is less effective than medium-intensity exercise. This is because when it is very intense, exercise becomes anaerobic, so you use up energy stores in muscles instead of fat.

If aerobic exercise is carried out continuously over a period of time some changes to the body occur. The heart becomes stronger. The amount of blood it can pump with each beat increases, which means that its rate slows down. This is good. Also, new blood vessels grow in the arms and legs. Existing blood vessels get bigger and stronger. This decreases the blood pressure and makes exercise easier as the oxygen-carrying capacity of those areas increases. Breathing also becomes easier. It is not possible to make the lungs work better, but if the rest of the cardio-vascular system is working more efficiently, you do not need to breathe as fast whatever you do.

Strength

Muscular strength is the ease with which the muscle is moved. Muscular endurance is the ability to continue to perform that work over time. If the muscle is not used it shrinks. This is called atrophy. If the muscle is exercised it grows. This is called hypertrophy. When a muscle grows the size of each individual cell grows. The number of cells remains the same. Improvements in muscular strength cause the body to burn more calories even at rest. Muscle is a metabolically active tissue. The more it is used the more calories are burned. In the context of cellulite, this is ideal because you are trying to burn fat. Over time if exercise is continued, muscle grows, it burns more fat, it tones and the overlying cellulite is depleted. Remember that spot fat reduction is not possible. The reason the cellulite is depleting is because the general level of fat in the body is depleting.

Another benefit of strength-training exercise is that muscular movement acts as a type of massage to the bony structures. When muscles are moved and used, bones are stimulated and become stronger and more dense. This can help to prevent osteoporosis.

Rest and recovery

Too much exercise is not good. Your body needs time to rest and recover. If you do not rest, your body will actually weaken.

Getting started

If you want to be successful with your fitness programme and want to feel good during and after exercise, you need to start in small increments of time and effort, and then increase gradually. This is where many people set themselves up to fail. They expect their body to perform activity at a level that is neither realistic nor recommended. After exercise they feel bad and then wrongly insist that it is the exercise itself that makes them feel worse.

When you begin an exercise programme, you should be gentle with your body. If you start slowly, your body will respond favourably, reinforcing the positive effects of your new exercise programme.

What type of exercise should you choose?

There are a number of factors to be considered when choosing a form of exercise. I said earlier in the chapter that most people choose the gym. This does not have to be the case. Also, what should you do once you are a member of the gym? Consider the following:

- time allotted for exercise

- alone or in a group

- indoors or outdoors

- variety

- skilled or non-skilled

- cost

- doctor's orders

- your age.

Create your own exercise chart

You should exercise at aerobic intensity levels of 60 to 90 per cent of maximum heart rate. Maximum recommended heart rate is, as mentioned earlier, 220 minus your age in years. If you are just starting an exercise programme you will begin exercising at the lower levels of heart rate. Once your body has adapted to that level you can then progress slowly and gradually into higher levels if desired. Your goal is to match up your current level of fitness with the appropriate intensity levels or zones of exercise. These levels are described subsequently.

For example, exercising at 60 per cent of your maximum heart rate may seem to require very little effort but it will still benefit your cardio-vascular system. It also burns a high percentage of fat as fuel. However, it requires more time to burn the calorific equivalent of exercising at a higher intensity level.

You can make your own training chart. Use the formula 220 minus your age to estimate maximum heart rates. For example, if you are 40, then your maximum heart rate when you are exercising should be 220 minus 40, which is 180 beats per minute.

Maximum heart rate is the highest number of heartbeats in 1 minute no matter how intense or prolonged the exercise stress.

Level 1 is when you exercise with your heart rate at 50 to 60 per cent of your estimated maximum heart rate. To find this level in beats per minute multiply your maximum heart rate by 0.5 or 0.6. If you are 40, your Level 1 heart rate is 90–108 beats per minute. Level 1 activity is very easy to sustain. Risk of injury is low. This is the best place to start an exercise programme.

Level 2 is exercising at 60–70 per cent of your estimated maximum heart rate. This is good for exercising at the beginning of a fitness programme or is a good warm-up for people who are very fit.

Level 3 is the aerobic zone. This is 70–80 per cent of the estimated maximum heart rate and is the place where fitness and aerobic efficiency occurs. Intensity is medium or may be quite difficult. You get fit very quickly at this level. Rest days must be included at this stage. Risk of muscle injury increases slightly.

Level 4 is 80–90 per cent of the estimated maximum heart rate. This level builds fitness and performance. It is hard and challenging. This level of exercise is still aerobic. Since fat can only burn in the presence of oxygen, you will not burn as high a percentage of fat as in the lower zones but you are burning plenty of calories.

Level 5 is 90–100 per cent of the estimated maximum heart rate. This level of exercise is not recommended for very long or for more than once or twice a week. This level of training is anaerobic. This means you need more than oxygen to sustain the muscles so the body has to change slightly from a metabolic point of view and give the muscles a helping hand by producing lactic acid. Used in interval training this level of exercise will help to increase fitness. Very little fat, mostly glucose, is burned at this intensity. The risk of muscle injury is at its highest here.

Your **fitness plan**, for someone concerned about the appearance of their cellulite, whatever exercise you are doing, could look like this:

Level 1 – 5 minutes

Level 2 – 5 minutes

Level 3 – 5 minutes

Level 4 – 5 minutes

Level 3 – 5 minutes

Level 2 – 5 minutes

Level 1 – 5 minutes

The benefits of exercise

A typical moderate exercise is walking briskly at about 6 km/h (4 m.p.h.). Exercises of greater intensity include swimming, racket sports such as tennis, and keep fit or aerobics exercises.

Exercise requiring mainly stamina is carried out through aerobic activities, such as running and swimming. These exercise the large muscle groups at a level that is not too intense to keep up for 20 minutes or more: for example, a run rather than a sprint. This type of exercise increases the demand on the oxygen-carrying capacity of heart, lungs and circulation, which gradually adapt and give greater endurance. This is beneficial to the appearance of cellulite.

Suppleness and strength improve the ability to carry out daily activities, and exercise in moderation can help prevent disability, especially as people get older. Exercise also contributes to balance and co-ordination, which in turn may help to prevent injury from falls, and other injuries. Strong muscles also give a firm, slim appearance.

Exercise is now widely valued for its capacity to instil a feeling of well-being; as well as boosting energy output, it discharges mental stress and physical tension and improves self-esteem. It has been claimed that exercise can reduce anxiety by distracting the mind from problems. All this is far more likely to happen if the chosen form of exercise is enjoyable in itself.

A major research programme carried out in the US in the 1990s concluded that people who take regular aerobic exercise acquire some protection against coronary heart disease, high blood pressure, diabetes mellitus, osteoporosis (fragile bones), bowel cancer and depression. There is also evidence that low levels of activity are associated with markedly increased death rates from a range of diseases. Increased activity, even in middle age, reduces that risk further.

Aerobic training also measurably reduces risk factors such as obesity (when combined with healthy dietary habits); lowered immunity; high levels of blood cholesterol, particularly low-density lipoproteins; high blood fat levels; thrombosis; and irregular heart rhythms.

Although research found that a high level of fitness was not necessary to gain most of these health benefits, some moderate exercise was regarded as far better than none. The results indicated that exercise was best taken in sessions as short as eight minutes, rather than all in one long session. These two conclusions are leading to the setting of new, more modest, targets for public health campaigns worldwide.

To reach a satisfactory level of health, it is thought that a total of at least 20 minutes per day, most days, of moderate exercise, or, alternatively, enough exercise to burn around 200 calories (837 joules) a day, is required. This total can be built up from several short sessions. Regular exercise is preferable to occasional intense sessions. It therefore helps to choose something that is enjoyable, and that can blend into daily life. Typical activities are walking and cycling instead of using a car, and using the stairs instead of taking the lift. It has been recommended that young people, particularly, should aim to do more than the minimum amount of exercise.

Calories burned during exercise

Calories per hour per lb body weight

Badminton	2.5	Rowing	3.0
Cycling	2.5	Skiing	3.5
Dancing	2.5	Squash	4.0
Golf	2.0	Swimming	3.5
Heavy gardening	3.0	Tennis	2.0
Hiking	3.5	Walking	3.5
House cleaning	1.5	Weight training	2.0
Jogging	4.0		

Types of training

Walking

BENEFITS

Walking is beneficial to people of all ages. It is free and no particular equipment is needed. It can be done anywhere, at any time.

It burns 3.5 calories per hour, per pound of body weight. If you weigh 200 lb, which is about 14 stone, you will burn about 700 calories per hour from a brisk walk. Sounds like a lot, but it is true.

RISK

There is no risk to the body unless you are walking about eight hours per day. Some people might find walking either boring or too time-consuming.

CELLULITE

In terms of cellulite a brisk walk is one of the best exercises. If you can get the heart rate up to 60 per cent of its calculated maximum, then you are at maximum fat burning capacity. If you are 40 years old then your estimated maximum heart rate should be 220 minus 40 which is 180. Sixty per cent of that is 108. This is not a hard rate to achieve through walking. At this heart rate, the said 40-year-old would have the best chance of reducing the appearance of their cellulite from walking.

PLAN FOR STARTING WALKING

Easy. Leave the house and just go. No warm-up is needed for a starter walker. Walk as far and as fast as is comfortable.

Jogging/running

BENEFITS

There are many benefits from jogging. If, again, you can get the heart rate quite low, below 140, then plenty of fat will be burned from this activity. There is more chance of toning the muscles of the bottom and legs from this type of exercise than from any other if you become proficient at it. After time you will develop a strong heart, more efficient lungs and beautifully toned thighs.

RISK

If you start jogging and you feel like you are dying then you are not ready for it. Get some brisk walking done first. Then run for a minute and walk some more, and so on until you are running for five minutes three or four times during a walk. That is the time to go for a slow jog. The distance and speed can be built up from that point over time. If you do not do this you have a very good chance of damaging the joints, especially if you are overweight and have not exercised for years.

You need a good warm-up as well. For beginners this involves walking for some time, then stretching, then starting the jog. Cold muscles do not like being stretched. Not doing this increases the risk of joint damage. If you damage the joints they will probably recover but it means you cannot exercise for some time while they rest.

If you only jog once a week it has been proven that your risk of heart disease is actually greater than if you do no exercise. This is because the heart has to get used to what you are doing. If you do not do enough then the heart never has time to grow with the exercise.

CELLULITE

Jogging to get rid of cellulite is an excellent idea if you

combine it with other methods. It allows you to burn fat and to tone the thighs and bottom. By the time you can jog for 30 minutes on a regular basis without stopping, you are a very fit person.

PLAN FOR STARTING RUNNING

Spend some weeks walking and running intermittently until you get to the stage where you can run for 30 minutes. The main emphasis on any jogging or running is not to hurt the joints. In time they will become stronger and you will be able to run further. Pushing yourself too hard at the start could mean that you need a year off jogging after you have only been doing it for three months.

You do not need much of a plan to jog. Be patient, and be constantly aware of your joints. Even if you do not push yourself you find that the results come surprisingly fast. Once you get over the initial two months where it is a drag to go out when it is cold, your life changes.

Cycling

BENEFITS

The benefits of cycling are cardio-vascular fitness, weight loss, loss of cellulite and that great feeling you get from exercising outside. It is a sport that can be done with all the family, with all the age groups.

There are a lot of cycling clubs out there as well. It is ideal for meeting other people, which will encourage you to carry on cycling.

RISK

Cycling in heavy traffic can be dangerous. Be aware of the road traffic and make sure you wear bright clothing. There are no risks to health from cycling unless you do massive amounts of it.

CELLULITE

Cycling is great for cellulite. It uses a lot of muscles, and a lot of energy. Fat is burned at an optimal rate because it is difficult to go very fast all the time on a bike. You end up with the heart pumping at about 60 per cent of its maximum, the fat burning range.

The legs where the cellulite is are toned and the amount of muscle there grows, tightening all the tissue.

PLAN FOR STARTING CYCLING

Go to one of those spinning classes in a gym, where a group of people get together in a room with a load of exercise bikes in it to cycle together. If you like it you can buy a bicycle. Remember to warm up.

Swimming

BENEFITS

Swimming is ideal for fat burning because once again it is very likely that you will end up exercising in the fat burning range. Swimming uses all the muscles in the body so it is excellent for general toning.

RISK

It can be difficult to swim effectively if a lot of other people are in the pool.

CELLULITE

Swimming will help you to burn fat but unless you push your self to breaking point every time you do it then swimming is not as specific for cellulite as some other exercises. This is because it is low impact. This means that the body weight is supported while exercising. Kicking the legs in a pool will not have the same benefits as pounding them on a road in terms of musclue tone. There is less chance that the joints will be damaged though.

PLAN FOR STARTING SWIMMING

Go to the swimming pool and swim as far as you can. Increase it every time you go. Swimming is the type of exercise where you can do this. Remember, though, that if you are already suffering from an illness, swimming is still hard exercise so check with your doctor.

Stair climber

This is fantastic for getting rid of cellulite. It targets all the right muscles to tone the legs and bottom. It is easy to attach yourself to a heart rate monitor while on it and to exercise in the fat burning range. Remember, you have to bend your legs or you are doing all the movement with the hips and the lower back. Plus, you are conning yourself into thinking that you are fitter than you actually are. If not done properly you may wonder why the cellulite is still there but you have a pain in your lower back and hips.

Ski machine

Again, very good for cellulite because it targets all the right muscles and allows you to monitor your heart rate. It is also impossible to do this exercise wrong because it will not move if you do not move, not like the stepper that allows small steps to be made. The workout on a ski machine is determined by the machine, which will only move in one way, exactly the same each revolution.

Rowing machine

This is a very hard workout. It is very difficult to do this exercise properly. It is easy to get backache because of the position your back is put in. It encourages the back to be in a pretty deformed position for the duration of the workout. When you get fitter and start to push yourself on this machine it is then that the injuries could start to occur. People train for years to learn the correct technique for rowing and to protect the back as much as possible. If this exercise must be done, build it up very gradually over years, not months.

Elliptical trainer (stepper with rolling feet)

An excellent exercise. It is medium impact, which means that it is not so hard on the joints, but you can still build up some excellent tone in the lower body.

It is impossible to do this exercise wrong because, once moving, it can only be done one way.

Aerobics classes

Aerobics provide a good workout for anybody of any standard as long as you can master the moves. It is also fun and provides an all-over body workout.

Because classes tend to be dominated by women, the emphasis of a lot of the exercise tends to be on the thighs, the bottom and the stomach. It is all medium-impact exercise. The joints are protected but there is a good chance that such a class will do a lot for the cellulite.

Step aerobics

More specific for the areas of cellulite. I have tried step aerobics and it is harder than it looks. Regular attendance will tone the lower body and help the appearance of cellulite.

Laugh when it gets hard

When the exercise becomes difficult, laugh. When your legs hurt, just laugh. This detracts from the discomfort and makes you push yourself a bit harder. It really works.

◆

CHAPTER EIGHTEEN

Detoxification

THIS CHAPTER IS VERY important in any book on cellulite. In other cellulite books you will read that detoxification is part of the plan to reduce the appearance of cellulite. I want to argue that detoxification has nothing to do with cellulite at all.

Misconceptions about toxins and cellulite

There are some common misconceptions surrounding toxins and cellulite that I am sure most people have heard. Some of them are as follows:

- cellulite occurs because all the rubbish in the body is pushed into the extremities and shows up as cellulite

- skin-brushing will help to rid cellulite of toxins

- improving the flow of lymph in cellulite will help to relieve it of its toxins

- drinking plenty of water will help to clear toxins away from cellulite

- a five-day detox plan will flush the system of toxins.

None of these are true. They are just not true. Consider the following questions:

- If cellulite occurred because all the toxins were pushed to the extremities, why do men not get cellulite?

- If skin-brushing got rid of the toxins in cellulite, why does skin-brushing have no effect on cellulite?

- If improving the flow of lymph in the cellulite helped to relieve it of its toxins, does this suggest that women have a worse flow of lymph than men?

- If drinking plenty of water helps to clear away the toxins from cellulite, why are so many of the treatments on sale for cellulite sold as substances that drain water away from cellulite?

- If we have proof of one thing concerning water and cellulite, it is that cellulite contains *more* water than ordinary fat.

- If a five-day detox plan will flush the system of toxins, does this suggest that men do not have any toxins in their body? After all, men do not tend to get cellulite.

In Chapter 1, I said that cellulite is made up of fat, collagen, proteoglycans and water. Nothing else. No toxins. I challenge anyone to tell me one single toxin that is in cellulite. There are none. There is no disputing this because cellulite has been looked at with a powerful microscope under the most rigorous medical testing criteria. No toxins were found.

Detoxification

It is difficult to define what is meant by 'detoxification'. Wherever it is mentioned in any literature or when it is talked about, nobody seems to know what 'toxins' are. Have you read any of the following?

• Toxins sometimes referred to without any explanation of what they are.

• They are sometimes said to be synthetic chemicals, pesticides, petroleum products, agro-chemicals, food additives or cleaning products.

• Toxins are said to be the waste that our body makes that is excreted via the kidneys, liver, bowel and skin.

Definitions

Detoxification to most people is stopping the consumption of some or all of the following:

○ cigarettes

○ alcohol

○ processed food

○ recreational drugs

○ fast food

○ fatty food

○ anything else that might make you feel unwell.

That abstinence is then often followed by:

a radical change in the diet to organic, grilled and boiled food with no salt

○ warm baths

○ going out for a walk

○ skin-brushing

○ cold showers

○ vigorous exercise

○ relaxation

○ yoga

○ anything else that might do you good.

Detoxification, then, is going on a diet, eating healthily and stopping ingesting anything that is considered naughty. Detoxification might also involve breathing cleaner air or going to bed earlier. It seems to be anything that will reduce the perceived level of poisons or toxins in the body.

A healthy liver will manage very well on a sensible diet without too much alcohol. Even so, anything that is perceived as detoxification will surely do no harm unless it is a period of prolonged starvation.

A short detoxification programme can result in an increased feeling of well-being. This seems to be related to detoxification of and by the liver.[1] Such detoxification would include eating simpler foods and drinking a lot of water. There might even be some exercise involved. It is certain, though, that such a programme would have no effect on cellulite unless it resulted in weight loss. The weight loss would improve the appearance of cellulite, not the detoxification.

Understanding detoxification

The best description of detoxification I can come up with is as follows. This is based on the accurate definition of a toxin as something that is potentially harmful, and so must be degraded by the liver before it is allowed into the bloodstream.

If a substance is not water soluble it cannot be excreted in the urine, and must be made water soluble by the liver to be excreted. Non-water soluble substances are one definition of a toxin.

Another definition of a toxin is a substance that the body has not encountered before, such as an unusual food additive, where the liver has to be used to excrete it. This is because there is not already a mechanism in place to get rid of it as it has never been ingested by the body before.

Elimination systems in the body

Lungs – the lungs eliminate carbon dioxide, which is a waste product. It is removed every time you breathe out. The only situations where there is too much carbon dioxide in the body are when a person has smoked for about 50 years. By this time the patient will be very ill all the time and will be spending a lot of time in hospital.

Lymph – is a fluid which takes away the waste products of metabolism in the tissues of the body. Via the lymphatic system these products are deposited in the bloodstream to be dealt with by the liver and the kidneys. Whatever you eat, you will still produce these waste products of metabolism.

Intestines – the intestines get rid of the bits of food that we cannot digest, such as fibre. There is a lot of bacteria in the faeces. This is normal. Without the bacteria we cannot digest the food properly. The reason that the faeces of a baby do not smell is because there are no bacteria in them. Because there are no bacteria in a baby's intestine, it has to live off milk for the first four months of its life because it cannot digest anything else. The gut is also involved in detoxification.[2] This is achieved by complex chemical reactions. Another way that the gut is involved in detoxification is that the bacteria that it contains can produce compounds that either induce or inhibit detoxification activities.

Liver – the liver is responsible for making chemicals safe. Anything that is poisonous in the body, such as alcohol, can hopefully be degraded by the liver into chemicals that are less harmful until a point comes when it can all be excreted from the body by the kidneys.

Kidneys – via the urine, the kidneys take away excess chemicals from the body. Most of these chemicals are made by the body or are needed by the body for life. The kidneys balance the amounts of these chemicals by retaining or excreting them. They also excrete a substance called urea, which is poisonous if you have too much of it, but it is a natural by-product of the metabolism that is essential for life.

Research

There are no research papers on detoxification and cellulite. Apart from the above, detoxification is eliminating from the system anything you have decided to eliminate.

There is a lot of research, though, to say what the structure of cellulite is at a molecular level and to show that there is nothing at all in cellulite that could be called a toxin.

Cellulite detoxification

In the context of cellulite, toxins can be considered to be the following:

○ fats in the food

○ a sedentary lifestyle

○ a poor diet.

Apart from the above, nothing else should be considered a toxin when trying to get rid of cellulite. The available research on what cellulite actually is, is quite solid. There is little evidence that cellulite is made of anything other than fats, connective tissue, proteoglycans and water. Water cannot be eliminated from the diet, and proteoglycans and connective tissue are there genetically. Fats are therefore the only things that can be eliminated from the diet because the rest of the constituents of cellulite will be there, whatever you do.

PART SIX

A Plan for the Elimination of Cellulite

◆

CHAPTER NINETEEN

Cellulite Treatments that Work and Those That Don't

THERE ARE SO MANY treatments available for the treatment of cellulite that it is difficult to pick the ones that are worth a try. In this chapter I visit the cellulite treatments that have been proven to work by clinical research and have been proven to work with good results. All these have been tested on a great many patients under the strictest supervision. I must stress here, though, that although these treatments undoubtedly work for cellulite it does not mean they are safe. They may be relatively safe, for example liposuction, but the risks still have to be looked at when considering any of these treatments.

Diet changes, exercise and endermologie can all be undertaken with a good assurance that they will not cause side-effects if carried out properly. As mentioned in Chapter 6, human growth hormone is a powerful substance with many effects. It seems excessive to use it just for cellulite when it has so many other actions.

There are other treatments that will probably work for cellulite but that are too difficult to test or have not been tested yet. These are presented in Chapter 23.

Just because the treatments in this chapter have been proven to work does not mean that they should be used. Some of them may be inaccessible to many people. Some may be wrong for you. It is a question of looking at the evidence and making a choice from the treatments that will work for cellulite and which are safe.

There are five treatments for cellulite that work undoubtedly. Only five. All the rest of the cellulite treatments that exist may or may not work, and the evidence to support them is not able to stand up to everybody's scrutiny. The five listed below do work. It cannot be denied that they work by any authority.

The only treatments for cellulite that work under everybody's scrutiny:

- **surgery**

- **diet**

- **exercise**

- **endermologie**

- **human growth hormone.**

Conclusion

Having looked at most of the existing treatments available for cellulite it is interesting that the ones that have been proven to work are simple, cheap and safe, with the exceptions of human growth hormone and surgery. This suggests that getting rid of your cellulite does not have to cost a lot of money.

The best of the cellulite treatments that will probably work

Below I have selected the cellulite treatments that have the most potential. These are all chosen from the end of each chapter in the book where the substances with the best chance of having a beneficial effect on cellulite have been listed.

The best of the cellulite treatments that will probably work are as follows:

- juniper
- kelp
- salmon oil
- omega-3
- ginger
- senna
- lecithin
- aminophylline
- retinoids
- skilled massage
- Ayurvedic medicine
- body wrap
- sunbathing.

◆

CHAPTER TWENTY

A Strict Plan for the Elimination of Cellulite

HAVING LOOKED AT MOST of the available treatments for cellulite, here is a plan for the reduction of cellulite.

Five of the substances in this chapter are known to work (see Chapter 19). The other 13 will probably work (see Chapter 19), but are not as proven as the top five substances.

The easiest way to start your elimination plan is to look at your diet. This can be integrated with some exercise. Then you should attend a good beautician. Undertaking those three things, diet, exercise and visiting a beautician, should lead to the effective reduction of the appearance of cellulite.

A one-week diet plan

Foods for the week

Breakfast, lunch and dinner for each day with calorific values for breakfast and lunch. Dinner recipes can be found in Chapter 16.

Monday	Yoghurt and fruit	**300**
	Potato soup, 2 slices of bread and large salad	**400**
	Baked seasoned salmon (8 cellulite specific ingredients)	
Tuesday	Scrambled eggs with potato and fruit	**300**
	Chicken breast with lettuce, tomato and fruit	**400**
	Japanese salad (5 cellulite specific ingredients)	
Wednesday	Toast, yoghurt and strawberries	**300**
	Hamburger, salad and fruit	**400**
	Italian pasta (2 cellulite specific ingredients)	
Thursday	Bread roll, orange juice, skimmed milk	**350**
	French onion soup and salad	**200**
	Lump crab and seaweed salad with fried rice noodles (2 cellulite specific ingredients)	
Friday	Shredded Wheat, skimmed milk, strawberries	**300**
	Tuna sandwich	**250**
	Orange chicken (3 cellulite specific ingredients)	
Saturday	Omelette (1 egg), orange, skimmed milk	**400**
	Spaghetti with tomato sauce and salad	**300**
	Ginger-flavoured stir-fried chicken (3 cellulite specific ingredients)	
Sunday	Boiled egg with toast and grapefruit	**350**
	Salad Nicoise and fruit	**350**
	Spicy fish curry (10 cellulite specific ingredients)	

Other activities

Suggestions only; others can be tried using the book as a reference to see if they work or not.

Monday	20 minutes' cardio-vascular workout (heart rate about 130)
Tuesday	Beautician's for a body wrap
Wednesday	20 minutes' cardio-vascular workout (heart rate about 130)
Thursday	Beautician's for endermologie
Friday	20 minutes' cardio-vascular workout (heart rate about 130)
Saturday	Massage
Sunday	No exercise or treatments

Following a weekly plan such as the one above will result in a rapid reduction in the appearance of your cellulite. All the food and activities listed have been shown to have an effect on cellulite.

◆

CHAPTER TWENTY-ONE

The Future of Cellulite Treatment

THROUGHOUT THE BOOK YOU will have read of treatments that should not be used yet as there is not enough research. Or you will have read that substances will probably work for the treatment of cellulite, but that they have not been formally proven as yet.

As with any field involving the body it is imperative that research from the manufacturer is demanded. Pills for cellulite are not taken for health reasons, but for vanity. Therefore, these cellulite treatments are not necessary and are not subject to mandatory research testing.

Once people become more safety conscious every company will have to provide research evidence for products sold that humans are ingesting. It is remarkable that anyone is prepared to swallow any pill they have bought over the internet.

> **The future of cellulite treatment is research into existing treatments.**

Future development

Possible areas for future development that would add to our knowledge of the causes of cellulite include the effects of androgens and oestrogens on it. Androgens are male hormones and oestrogens female. This would be done by examination of female adults and children who had too much male hormone, such as those who are born that way, and males with too little androgen, such as those with testicular feminisation.

The effects of male and female DNA on cellulite could be examined in adults and children with Turner syndrome (XXO), Klinefelter (XXY), or other such syndromes. These diseases are rare ones, where for instance a man is born as a man but has more female DNA in him than he should have. If such a man developed cellulite then this adds to the argument that cellulite is caused by a lack of testosterone. If a woman who was born with too much male DNA did not get cellulite then that adds to the argument that cellulite is caused by a lack of testosterone.

Children could be studied for the presence of cellulite at various stages of their growth to pinpoint the time at which cellulite starts to develop.

Lastly, the structure of the skin and circulating concentrations of male and female hormones should be examined in women who have cellulite and women who do not have cellulite to try to determine what the difference is between the two types.

It is not yet possible to completely cure cellulite.

All the available evidence now, if looked at together, suggests that the structure of cellulite should be studied to look for a cure. It is the collagen in the cellulite tissue that causes the majority of the problem and this is the part of the tissue that cannot be treated yet. If collagen could be strengthened, cellulite would be cured.

So far, the most promising treatments aimed at the collagen in the cellulite are based on surgery and chemicals targeting particular types of collagen in the tissue. There is still a very great deal of work to be done on the subject, though, to make it safe and successful.

As with most other types of medicine, a total cure will be possible one day. Until then, have fun with this book. Following the plans here will certainly reduce your cellulite as much as any other treatment combination you could find.

Useful Addresses

Action for the Victims of Medical Accidents
44 High Street
Croydon
CR0 1YB
020 8686 8333

Aromatherapy Organisations Council
PO Box 19834
London
SE25 6WF
020 8251 7912

Association of Reflexologists
27 Old Gloucester Street
London WC1 3XX
0870 5673320

Ayurvedic Medical Association UK
59 Dulverton Road
South Croydon CR2 8PJ
020 8682 3876

British Complementary Medicine Association
PO Box 2074
Seaford BN25 1HQ
0845 345 5977

British Homeopathic Association
15 Clerkenwell Close
London EC1R 0AA
020 7566 7800

London School of Aromatherapy
PO Box 32820
London N1 1GB
0800 716 847

National Institute of Medical Herbalists
56 Longbrook Street
Exeter EX4 6AH
01392 426022

Women's Nutritional Advisory Service
PO Box 268
Lewes
East Sussex BN7 2QN
(01273) 487366

Shiatsu Society
Eastlands Court
St Peters Road
Rugby CV21 3QP
01788 55051

Appendix I

Substances That Have No Rational Reason for Being Sold as Cellulite Treatments

The following is a list of substances that are all claimed to be treatments for cellulite. The fact that I say there is no evidence to support their use in this context does not mean they do not work. It means there are no trials on their use and no logic behind their use as cellulite treatments.

If a GP tried to give you a substance that had not been rigorously tested and which was not even supported by logic, would you take it?

Apple rind extract
Geranium
Hydrangea arborescens root
Citrus aurantium
Brolein
Papaya
Pepsin
L-carnatine and L-tartrate
Citrin
Gotu kola
Ferrous fumarate
Apple cider vinegar

Appendix II

Ingredients of Widely-used Cellulite Pills

Cellasene contains:

Bioflavanoids
Evening primrose oil
Ginger oleoresin
Ginkgo biloba
Gotu kola
Grape seed
Hawthorn
Horse chestnut
Juniper oil
Kelp
Salmon oil
Lecithin
Rosemary oil
Turmeric
Vitamin B6
Vitamin E
Yellow sweet clover

Cellu Rid contains:

Vitamin C
Iron
Herba cell (senna leaves, cascara sagrada bark, apple rind extract,

milk thistle root, piper nigrum (tailed pepper) extract, cinnamon root extract)
White willow bark
Kelp
Apple cider vinegar
Guarana seed
Lecithin
Rose hips
Buchu leaves
Couch grass
Hydrangea arborescens root
Uva ursi
Juniper berries

Actrim contains:

Brolein
Papaya
Pepsin
L-carnatine and L-tartrate
Chromium tri-picolinate

Cell pill contains:

Bladder wrack
Horsechestnut
Omega-3 fatty acids
GLA
Gotu kola
Grape seed extract
Ginkgo biloba

References

CHAPTER 1

1. Rosenbaum, M. and Hellmer, J. (1998) An exploratory investigation of the morphology and biochemistry of cellulite. *Plast Reconstr Surg*, **101**:7, 1934–9.
2. Pierard, G.E., Nizet, J.L. and Pierard-Franchimont, C. (2000) Cellulite, from standing fat herniation to hypodermal stretch marks. *Am J Dermatopathol*, **22**(1): 34–7.
3. Nurnberger, F. and Muller, G. (1978) So-called cellulite: an invented disease. *J Dermatol Surg Oncol*, **4**: 221.
4. Ibid.
5. Lotti, T. and Ghersetich, I. (1990) Proteoglycans in so-called cellulite. *Int J Dermatol*, **29**: 272.
6. Gruber, D.M. and Huber, J.C. (1999) Gender specific medicine: the new profile of gynaecology *Gynecol Endocrinol*, **13**(1): 1–6.
7. Pierard, G.E., Nizet, J.L. and Pierard-Franchimont, C. (2000) Cellulite, from standing fat herniation to hypodermal stretch marks. *Am J Dermatopathol*, **22**(1): 34–7.
8. Lotti, T., Ghersetich, I., Grappone, C. and Dini, G. (1990) Proteoglycans in so-called cellulite. *Int J Dermatol*, **29**(4): 272.
9. Curri, S.B. and Bombardelli, E. (1994) Local lipodystrophy and districtual microcirculation. *Cosmet*, **109**: 52–65.
10. Curri, S.B. (1993) Cellulite and fatty tissue micro-circulation. *Cosmet*, **108**: 51–8.

CHAPTER 2

1. Jones, S.M., Zhong, Z., Enomoto, N., Schemmer, P. and Thurman R.G. (1998) Dietary juniper berry oil minimizes hepatic reperfusion injury in the rat. *Hepatology*, **28**(4): 1042–50.

2. Sanchez de Medina, F., Gamez, M.J., Jimenez, I., Jimenez, J., Osuna, J.I. and Zarzuelo, A. (1994) Hypoglycemic activity of juniper 'berries'. *Planta Med*, 60(3): 197–200.

3. Ibid.

4. Takacsova, M., Pribela, A. and Faktorova, M. (1995) Study of the anti-oxidative effects of thyme, sage, juniper and oregano. *Nahrung*, 39(3): 241–3.

5. Argento, A., Tiraferri, E. and Marzaloni, M. (2000) Oral anticoagulants and medicinal plants. An emerging interaction. *Ann Ital Med Int*, 15(2): 139–43.

6. Yan, X., Nagata, T. and Fan, X. (1998). Antioxidative activities in some common seaweeds. Plant Foods. *Hum Nutr*, 52(3): 253–62.

7. Leenen, R., Roodenburg, A.J., Tijburg, L.B. and Wiseman, S.A. (2000) A single dose of tea with or without milk increases plasma antioxidant activity in humans. *Eur J Clin Nutr*, 54(1): 87–92.

8. Hurrell, R.F., Reddy, M. and Cook, J.D. (1999) Inhibition of non-haem iron absorption in man by polyphenolic–containing beverages. *Br J Nutr*, 81(4): 289–95.

9. Micklefield, G.H., Greving, I. and May, B. (2000) Effects of peppermint oil and caraway oil on gastroduodenal motility. *Phytother Res*, 14(1): 20–3.

10. Venkataramanan, R., Ramachandran, V., Komoroski, B.J., Zhang, S., Schiff, P.L. and Strom, S.C. (2000) Milk thistle, a herbal supplement, decreases the activity of CYP3A4 and uridine diphosphoglucuronosyl transferase in human hepatocyte cultures. *Drug Metab Dispos*, 28(11): 1270–3.

11. Bass, N.M. (1999) Is there any use for nontraditional or alternative therapies in patients with chronic liver disease? *Curr Gastroenterol Rep*, 1(1): 50–6.

12. Bagchi, D., Bagchi, M., Stohs, S.J., Das, D.K., Ray, S.D., Kuszynski, C.A. *et al.* (2000) Free radicals and grape seed proanthocyanidin extract: importance in human health and disease prevention. *Toxicology*, 148(2–3): 187–97.

13. Benoni, H., Dallakian, P. and Taraz, K. (1996) Studies on the essential oil from guarana. *Z Lebensm Unters Forsch*, 203(1): 95–8.

14. Burits, M. and Bucar, F. (2000) Antioxidant activity of nigella sativa essential oil. *Phytother Res*, 14(5): 323–8.

15. Greenberg, S. and Frishman, W.H. (1990) Co-enzyme Q10: a new drug for cardiovascular disease. Bio-energetical and free radical scavenger properties. *J Clin Pharmacol*, 30(7): 596–608.

16. Powers, S.K. and Lennon, S.L. (1999) Analysis of cellular responses to free radicals: focus on exercise and skeletal muscle. *Proc Nutr Soc*, 58(4): 1025–33.

17. Koul, I.B. and Kapil, A. (1993) Evaluation of the liver protective potential of piperine, an active principle of black and long peppers. *Planta Med*, 59(5): 417–17.

18. Singh, A. and Rao A.R. (1993) Evaluation of the modulatory influence of black pepper (Piper nigrum, L.) on the hepatic detoxification system. *Cancer Lett*, **72**(1-2): 5-9.

19. Friedman, M., Kozukue, N. and Harden, L.A. (2000) Cinnamaldehyde content in foods determined by gas chromatography-mass spectrometry. *J Agric Food Chem*, **48**(11): 5702-9.

20. Shobana, S. and Naidu, K.A. (2000) Antioxidant activity of selected Indian spices. Prostaglandins. *Leukot Essent Fatty Acids*, **62**(2): 107-10.

21. Asai, A., Nakagawa, K. and Miyazawa, T. (1999) Antioxidative effects of turmeric, rosemary and capsicum extracts on membrane phospholipid peroxidation and liver lipid metabolism in mice. *Biosci Biotechnol Biochem*, **63**(12): 2118-22.

22. Selvam, R., Subramanian, L., Gayathri, R. and Angayarkanni, N. (1995) The anti-oxidant activity of turmeric (Curcuma longa). *J Ethnopharmacol*, **47**(2): 59-67.

CHAPTER 3
1. Harris, W.S., Connor, W.E. and McMurry, M.P. (1983) The comparative reductions of the plasma lipids and lipoproteins by dietary polyunsaturated fats: salmon oil versus vegetable oils. *Metabolism*, **32**(2): 179-84.

2. O'Keefe, J.H. Jr, and Harris, W.S. (2000) From Inuit to implementation: omega-3 fatty acids come of age. *Mayo Clin Proc*, **75**(6): 607-14.

3. Weber, P. and Raederstorff, D. Triglyceride-lowering effect of omega-3 LC-polyunsaturated fatty acids - a review. *Nutr Metab Cardiovasc Dis*, **10**(1): 28-37.

4. Santamarina-Fojo, S., Lambert, G., Hoeg, J.M. and Brewer, H.B. Jr. (2000) Lecithin-cholesterol acyltransferase: role in lipoprotein metabolism, reverse cholesterol transport and atherosclerosis. *Curr Opin Lipidol*, **11**(3): 267-75.

5. Press, R.I., Geller, J. and Evans, G.W. (1990) The effect of chromium picolinate on serum cholesterol and apolipoprotein fractions in human subjects. *West J Med*, **152**(1): 41-5.

6. Howes, J.B., Sullivan, D., Lai, N., Nestel, P., Pomeroy, S., West, L. *et al.* (2000) The effects of dietary supplementation with isoflavones from red clover on the lipoprotein profiles of post-menopausal women with mild to moderate hypercholesterolaemia. *Atherosclerosis*, **152**(1): 143-7.

7. Chen, J.D., Wu, Y.Z., Tao, Z.L., Chen, Z.M. and Liu, X.P. (1995) Hawthorn (shan zha) drink and its lowering effect on blood lipid levels in humans and rats. *World Rev Nutr Diet*, **77**: 147-54.

CHAPTER 4

1. Ernst, E. (1999) Herbal medications for common ailments in the elderly. *Drugs Aging*, 15(6): 423–8.
2. Pittler, M.H. and Ernst, E. (1998) Horse-chestnut seed extract for chronic venous insufficiency. A criteria-based systematic review. *Arch Dermatol*, 134(11): 1356–60.
3. Greeske, K. and Pohlmann, B.K. (1996) Horse chestnut seed extract – an effective therapy principle in general practice. Drug therapy of chronic venous insufficiency. *Fortschr Med*, 114(15): 196–200.
4. Bascaglia, D.A. and Conte, E.T. The treatment of cellulite with methyl xanthine and herbal extract based cream: an ultrasonographic analysis.
5. Bray, G.A. (1999) Drug treatment of obesity. *Baillieres Best Pract Res Clin Endocrinol Metab*, 13(1): 131–48.
6. Pittler, M.H. and Ernst, E. (2000) Ginkgo biloba extract for the treatment of intermittent claudication: a meta-analysis of randomized trials. *Am J Med*, 108(4): 276–81.
7. Diamond, B.J., Shiflett, S.C., Feiwel, N., Matheis, R.J. Noskin, O., Richards, J.A. *et al.* (2000) Ginkgo biloba extract: mechanisms and clinical indications. *Arch Phys Med Rehabil*, 81(5): 668–78.
8. Bucci, L.R. (2000) Selected herbals and human exercise performance. *Am J Clin Nutr*, 72(2 Suppl): 624S–36S.
9. Hou, J.P. (1977) The chemical constituents of ginseng plants. *Comp Med East West*, 5(2): 123–45.
10. Ong, Y.C. and Yong, E.L. (2000) Panax (ginseng) – panacea or placebo? Molecular and cellular basis of its pharmacological activity. *Ann Acad Med Singapore*, 29(1). 42–6.
11. Nocerino, E., Amato, M. and Izzo, A.A. (2000) The aphrodisiac and adaptogenic properties of ginseng. *Fitoterapia*, 71 Suppl 1: S1–S5.
12. Miller, L.G. (1998) Herbal medicinals: selected clinical considerations focusing on known or potential drug-herb interactions. *Arch Intern Med*, 158(20): 2200–11.

CHAPTER 5

1. Micklefield, G.H., Redeker, Y., Meister V., Jung, O., Greving, I., and May, B. (1999) Effects of ginger on gastroduodenal motility. *Int J Clin Pharmacol Ther*, 37(7):341–6
2. Ahmed, R.S., and Sharma, S.B. (1997) Biochemical studies on combined effects of garlic (Allium sativum Linn) and ginger (Zingiber officinale Rosc) in albino rats. *Indian J Exp Biol*; 35(8):841–3.
3. Langner, E., Greifenberg, S., and Gruenwald, J. (1998) Ginger: history and use. *Adv Ther*, 15(1):25–44.

4. Epstein, M.T., Espiner, E.A., Donald, R.A. and Hughes, H. (1977) Effect of eating liquorice on the renin-angiotensin aldosterone axis in normal subjects. *Br Med J*, **1**(6059): 488–90.

5. Olukoga, A. and Donaldson, D.J.R. (2000) Liquorice and its health implications. *Soc Health*, **120**(2): 83–9.

6. Swanston-Flatt, S.K., Day, C., Bailey, C.J. and Flatt, P.R. (1989) Evaluation of traditional plant treatments for diabetes: studies in streptozotocin diabetic mice. *Acta Diabetol Lat*, **26**(1): 51–5.

7. Beaux, D., Fleurentin, J. and Mortier, F. (1999) Effects of extracts of Orthosiphon stamineus Benth, Hieracium pilosella L., Sambucus nigra L. and Arctostaphylos uva-ursi (L.) Spreng. in rats. *Phytother Res*, **13**(3): 222–5.

8. Izzo, A.A., Sautebin, L., Rombola, L. and Capasso, F. (1997) The role of constitutive and inducible nitric oxide synthase in senna- and cascara-induced diarrhoea in the rat. *Eur J Pharmacol*, **323**(1): 93–7.

9. Lis-Balchin, M. and Hart, S. (1999) Studies on the mode of action of the essential oil of lavender. *Phytother Res*, **13**(6): 540–2.

CHAPTER 6

1. Butler, R.N., Fossel, M., Pan, C.X., Rothman, D.J. and Rothman, S.M. (2000) Anti-aging medicine. 2. Efficacy and safety of hormones and antioxidants. *Geriatrics*, **55**(7): 48–52, 55–6, 58.

2. Heffernan, M.A., Jiang, W.J., Thorburn, A.W. and Ng, F.M. (2000) Effects of oral administration of a synthetic fragment of human growth hormone on lipid metabolism. *Am J Physiol Endocrinol Metab* **279**(3): E501–7.

3. Gehring, W., Bopp, R., Rippke, F. and Gloor, M. (1999) Effect of topically applied evening primrose oil on epidermal barrier function in atopic dermatitis as a function of vehicle. *Arzneimittelforschung*, **49**(7): 635–42.

4. Burg, M.B. (1995) Molecular basis of osmotic regulation. *Am J Physiol*, **268**(6 Pt 2): F983–96.

CHAPTER 7

1. Bos, J.D. and Meinardi, M.M. (2000) The 500 Dalton rule for the skin penetration of chemical compounds and drugs. *Exp Dermatol* **9**(3): 165–9.

CHAPTER 8

1. Vogler, B.K. and Ernst, E. (1999) Aloe vera: a systematic review of its clinical effectiveness. *Br J Gen Pract*, **49**(447): 823–8.

2. Klein, A.D. and Penneys, N.S. (1988) Aloe vera. *J Am Acad Dermatol*, **18**(4 Pt 1): 714–20.

3. Frick, R.W. (2000) Three treatments for chronic venous insufficiency: escin, hydroxyethylrutoside, and Daflon. *Angiology*, **51**(3): 197–205.

4. Bauer, R. (1996) Echinacea drugs – effects and active ingredients. *Z Arztl Fortbild (Jena)*, **90**(2): 111–15.

5. Miller, L.G. (1998) Herbal medicinals: selected clinical considerations focusng on known or potential drug-herb interactions. *Arch Intern Med*, **158**(20): 2200–11.

CHAPTER 9

1. Collis, N. and Elliot, L.A. (1999) Cellulite treatment, a myth or reality: a prospective, randomized controlled trial of two therapies, endermologie and aminophylline cream. *Plast Reconst surg*, **104**(4): 1110–14.
2. Greenway, F.L. and Bray, G.A. (1987) Regional fat loss from the thighs of obese women after adrenergic modulation. *Clin Ther*, **9**: 663–9.
3. Hamilton, E.C., Greenway, F.L. and Bray, G.A. (1993) Regional fat loss from the thighs in women using topical 2% aminophylline cream. *Obesity Res*, **1**: 955.

CHAPTER 10

1. Illouz, Y.G. (1989) *Body Sculpturing by Lipoplasty*. Churchill Livingstone, Edinburgh.
2. Adamo, C., Mazzocchi, M., Rossi, A. and Scuderi, N. (1997) Ultrasonic liposculpturing: extrapolations from the analysis of in vivo sonicated adipose tissue. *Plast Reconst Surg*, **100**(1): 220–6.
3. Grotting, J.C. and Beckenstein, M.S. (1999) The solid probe technique in ultrasound assisted lipoplasty. *Clin Plast Surg*, **26**(2): 245–54; viii.
4. Mendes, F.H. (2000) External ultrasound-assisted lipoplasty from our own experience. *Aesthetic Plast Surg*, **24**(4): 270–4.
5. Gasparotti, M. (1992) Superficial liposuction. a new application for the technique for aged and flaccid skin. *Aesthetic Plast Surg*, **16**(2): 141–53.
6. Toledo, L.S. (1991) Syringe liposculpture: a two year experience. *Aesthetic Plast Surg*, **15**(4): 321–6.
7. Slim, K. (1999) Laparoscopic surgery for obesity. *J Chir (Paris)*, **136**(4): 188–97.
8. Fourtanier, G. and Cadiere, G.B. (1999) Surgery for pathological obesity. *Ann Chir Plast Esthet*, **44**(4): 431–9.

CHAPTER 11

1. Eliska, O. and Eliskova, M. (1995) Are peripheral lymphatics damaged by high pressure manual massage? *Lymphology*, **28**(1): 21–30.
2. Andersen, L., Hojris, I., Erlandsen, M. and Andersen, J. (2000) Treatment of breast-cancer-related lymphedema with or without manual lymphatic drainage – a randomized study. *Acta Oncol*, **39**(3): 399–405.
3. Chang, P., Wiseman, J., Jacoby, T., Salisbury, A.V. and Ersek, R.A. (1998) Noninvasive mechanical body contouring: (Endermologie) A one-year clinical outcome study update. *Aesthetic Plast Surg*, **22**(2): 145–53.

4. Marchand, J.P. and Privat, Y. (1991) A new instrumental method for the treatment of cellulite. *Medicine au Ferminin (French)*, **39**: 25–34.

5. Baumgartner, F.J., Pandya, A., Omari, B.O., Pandya, A., Turner, C., Milliken, J.C. *et al.* (1997) Ultrasonic debridement of mitral calcification. *J Card Surg*, **12**(4): 240–2.

6. Oh, D.H., Eulau, D., Tokugawa, D.A., McGuire, J.S. and Kohler, S. (1999) Five cases of calciphylaxis and a review of the literature. *J Am Acad Dermatol*, **40**(6 Pt 1): 979–87.

7. Vinge, O.D., Evardsen, L., Jensen, F.K., Lassen, F.G., Wernerman, J. and Kehlet, H. (1998) Effect of transcutaneous electric muscle stimulation on postoperative muscle mass and protein synthesis. *Ugeskr Laeger*, **160**(3): 283–6.

CHAPTER 12

1. Stephenson, N.L., Weinrich, S.P. and Tavakoli, A.S. (2000) The effects of foot reflexology on anxiety and pain in patients with breast and lung cancer. *Oncol Nurs Forum*, **27**(1): 67–72.

2. Sudmeier, I., Bodner, G., Egger, I., Mur, E., Ulmer, H. and Herold, M. (1999) Changes of renal blood flow during organ-associated foot reflexology measured by color Doppler sonography. *Forsch Komplementarmed*, **6**(3): 129–34.

3. White, A.R., Williamson, J., Hart, A. and Ernst, E. (2000) A blinded investigation into the accuracy of reflexology charts. *Complement Ther Med* **8**(3): 166–72.

CHAPTER 13

1. Cooke, B. and Ernst, E. (2000) Aromatherapy: a systematic review. *Br J Gen Pract*, Jun, **50**(455): 493–6.

2. Burkhard, P.R., Burkhardt, K., Haenggeli, C.A. and Landis, T. (1999) Plant-induced seizures: reappearance of an old problem. *J Neurol*, **246**(8): 667–70.

3. Hjelvik, M. and Morenskog, E. (1997) The principles of homeopathy. *Tidsskr Nor Laegeforen*, **117**(17): 2497–501.

4. Miller, L.G. (1998) Herbal medicinals: selected clinical considerations focusing on known or potential drug-herb interactions. *Arch Intern Med*, **158**(20): 2200–11.

CHAPTER 14

1. Bernstein, E.F., Underhill, C.B., Hahn, P.J., Brown, D.B. and Uitto, J. (1996) Chronic sun exposure alters both the content and distribution of dermal glycosaminoglycans. *Br J Dermatol*, **135**(2): 255–62.

2. Van Horn, L., Emidy, L.A., Liu, K.A., Liao, Y.L., Ballew, C., King, J. *et al.* (1988) Serum lipid response to a fat-modified, oatmeal-enhanced diet. *Prev Med*, **17**(3): 377–86.

3. Thune, P., Nilsen, T., Hanstad, I.K., Gustavsen, T., Lovig Dahl, H. (1988) The water barrier function of the skin in relation to the water content of stratum corneum, pH and skin lipids. The effect of alkaline soap and syndet on dry skin in elderly, non-atopic patients. *Acta Derm Venereol*, 68(4): 277–83.

4. Levi-Schaffer, F., Shani, J., Politi, Y., Rubinchik, E. and Brenner, S. (1996) Inhibition of proliferation of psoriatic and healthy fibroblasts in cell culture by selected Dead-sea salts. *Pharmacology*, 52(5): 321–8.

5. Sukenik, S., Neumann, L., Buskila, D., Kleiner-Baumgarten, A., Zimlichman, S., Horowitz, J. (1990) Dead Sea bath salts for the treatment of rheumatoid arthritis. *Clin Exp Rheumatol*, 8(4): 353–7.

6. Harari, M., Barzillai, R. and Shani, J. (1998) Magnesium in the management of asthma: critical review of acute and chronic treatments, and Deutsches Medizinisches Zentrum's (DMZ's) clinical experience at the Dead Sea. *J Asthma*, 35(7): 525–36.

CHAPTER 18

1. MacIntosh, A. and Ball, K. (2000) The effects of a short program of detoxification in disease-free individuals. *Altern Ther Health Med*, 6(4): 70–6.

2. DeAnn, J. and Liska, Ph.D. (1998) The detoxification enzyme systems. *Altern Med Rev*, 3(3): 187–98.

Index